FOOD FIT TO EAT

FOOD FIT TO EAT
How to survive processed food

Professor David M Conning
*Director-General, British Nutrition
Foundation*

Lis Leigh
Food Correspondent, The Sunday Times

Barry D Ricketts
Writer and Consultant

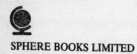

SPHERE BOOKS LIMITED

SPHERE BOOKS LTD

Published by the Penguin Group
27 Wrights Lane, London W8 5TZ, England
Viking Penguin Inc., 40 West 23rd Street, New York, New York 10010, USA
Penguin Books Australia Ltd, Ringwood, Victoria, Australia
Penguin Books Canada Ltd, 2801 John Street, Markham, Ontario, Canada L3R 1B4
Penguin Books (NZ) Ltd, 182–190 Wairau Road, Auckland 10, New Zealand

Penguin Books Ltd, Registered Offices: Harmondsworth, Middlesex, England

First published in Great Britain by Sphere Books Ltd, 1988

Produced on behalf of the
British Nutrition Foundation, 15 Belgrave Square, London SW1X 8PS, by
CORPORATE AFFAIRS
Amney House, Badgers Wood,
Farnham Common, Buckinghamshire

Printed and bound in Great Britain by
Richard Clay Ltd, Bungay, Suffolk

Contents

Preface

The perils of processed food have been much in the news in recent years. The term 'processed food' has been used to describe products containing additives, fast foods, snacks, any kind of packaged food, airline meals and virtually the whole range of confectionery. It has become clear that writers using the term seldom have much idea what it means and their reaction to it depends more on the kind of article they want to write than on processed food itself. A political harangue, a 'foodie' diatribe, a new concern (meaning an anxiety-creating idea) all use 'processed food' as the harridan in their particular witch-hunt.

In fact, the processing of food is among the oldest of human activities and without it we simply would not eat. But as human society becomes more industrialized and urbanized, so fewer of us appreciate what is needed to bring food from the field to the table.

At the British Nutrition Foundation, our main aim is to help the consumer understand about food and nutrition, and this book is an attempt to put the whole subject into some kind of perspective. Within its pages you will find all you need to know about food production and manufacture, nutrition and health, taste and convenience; the good and the bad. You will then be able to decide for yourself how food is going to figure in your life, confident that if you apply the lessons, you can make the right decisions. Personal compromises will be needed because everyone has different preferences, and when you are aiming at a balanced diet likes and dislikes do get in the way.

Try to read the whole book before dipping into chapters or topics. In this way you will get an overall view against which you can test your particular concern; and maybe you will find it's not such a concern any more. If you need to know more, write to us at the Foundation and we will try to help.

Above all, remember that eating should be enjoyable. Nature provides a wide variety of foods so that we will get all the nutrients we need. The only dangers arise from eating too much or eating too much of a particular type of food.

Ring the changes and you will be laughing all the way to the health bank.

Acknowledgements

The authors would like to thank all who contributed their thoughts and time to this book, including the academic and industrial advisers to the British Nutrition Foundation. Special thanks are due to Baxters of Speyside and the National Consumer Council for permission to reproduce material supplied, and to Professor A. W. Holmes of the British Food Manufacturing Industries Research Association and Marks & Spencer for specific comment.

The authors would also like to acknowledge the indispensable help of Richard Cottrell, Fiona Campbell, Gill Fine, Marnie Sommerville and Helen Merskey of the British Nutrition Foundation. Special thanks to Mary Ransom of the Foundation for her patience in typing (and retyping) the copy; and to Rhonda Smith of Corporate Affairs for diligent editing.

List of Illustrations

List of Tables

1 The Food Controversy

Food is a basic need and of interest to everyone.
Why is it the subject of such distortion, claim and
counterclaim? Danger! Vested interests at work.

Barry D Ricketts

The earliest cave paintings bear witness to the central role of food
in our hazardous and brutal beginnings. Throughout history, food
has been a symbolic thread which, with religion, has become woven
into people's cultural fabric. In all human society, from the most
primitive to the most advanced, food is more than mere fuel.

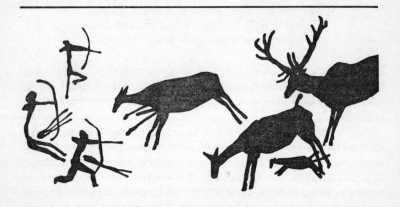

Food symbolism forms time-capsules in our language. The 'olive
branch' of peace reflects the cultivation of the olive during the time
of peace and stability which followed Roman conquest; 'sacred
cow' now means so much more than an animal revered by Hindus.

As civilization progressed, so attitudes towards food changed.
Frugality and abstinence were regarded as a mark of gentility in
Norman times; a century or so later, the rich were often gluttons.

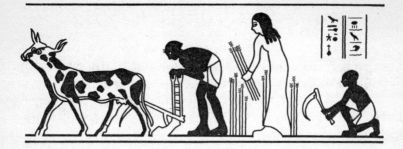

These trends were not just reflections of the availability of food, but had as much to do with lifestyles and badges of status.

The production, distribution, quality, taxation and availability of food have caused political upheaval and war throughout recorded history. The food supplier or processor has often been regarded with some suspicion. In his *Canterbury Tales*, Chaucer says of the miller:

> His was a master hand at stealing grain
> He felt it with his thumb and thus he knew
> Its quality and took three times his due.

This not only characterizes the guile of the miller, but indicates a general scepticism about those who hold powerful positions within the economics of food, a scepticism which has endured down the centuries.

People have suspected food to be harmful to health for almost as long as they have known it to be vital. Although tomatoes were available in Europe from the fifteenth century, they were unpopular in England until the beginning of the twentieth, as they were widely believed to be a cause of gout and cancer. Despite the Irish people's love of the potato, the English disdained the crop for home consumption until relatively recently, believing it to cause flatulence and even leprosy. The connection between diet and health has been recognized for centuries, and across cultures. In the sixteenth century, the physician Andrew Boorde wrote in his *Dyetary of Health*:

A good cook is half physician. For the chief Physic (the counsil of a physician excepted) doth come from the kitchen; wherefor the physician and cook must consult together for the preparation of meat ... For if the physician without the cook prepare any meat except he be very expert, he will make a worse dish of meat, that which the sick cannot take.

Our love–hate relationship with food and everything connected with it has persisted, and has never required rationality to fuel it. Today, our voracious media with an appetite for conflict and sensation provides a ready outlet for all manner of food and food-related topics. There is no shortage of material with which newspapers, magazines, radio and television programmes can bombard an ever more confused public.

By the same token, there is a rich literature on the subject, replenished almost weekly by new titles, proving that our intellectual appetite for facts about food is as demanding as our desire for new gastronomy and variety of products.

Today, food remains a source of conflict and division. Official and self-appointed health workers and agencies criticize the products and practices of the food industry and castigate government for under-regulation. Scientists and quasi-scientific journalists publish serious papers claiming ever-widening areas of correlation between diet and a plethora of serious diseases.

The food industry itself is divided and ambiguous on the subject, at one time defending a beleaguered foodstuff, at another, joining the chorus of criticism if it helps commercial success elsewhere.

Critics of the food industry and of production and distribution policies are frequently guilty of unscientific rationale. The authorities themselves lend credibility to the conspiracy theory by their reluctance to explain their actions.

The wide spectrum of food issues that have claimed public attention in recent years is evidence of the concern which surrounds human nutrition. It is also deeply worrying because it demonstrates that the state of popular knowledge about elementary nutrition is woefully inadequate.

This is the crisis confronting consumers, manufacturers and medical professionals alike, for it allows both deliberate and unintended abuse to flourish in our society, in a way that usurps the right of individuals to know what happens to their bodies when they eat.

Vested interests abound, some of them well-motivated, but all of them tending to obscure the picture. The result is that at a time when consumers are experiencing more choices, stresses and special dietary needs than ever before, they are confronted with political proselytizing, opportunistic advertising and bureaucratic double-talk.

Many organizations regularly publish advisory information to the general public, but little guidance on their background is available to the casual reader. The battleground for this daily war of misinformation is the public's health, and however well-intentioned some of the contributors to this controversy may be, it is time to call a halt. Public health is not an appropriate target for propaganda, whatever the cause.

Sadly, the present state of affairs could not have come about if public health had been given equal weight to national economic factors when successive governments planned agricultural and food-production policy. This position has arisen because science and medicine have not asserted their views (in some cases, have not developed views) about safe nutritional practices in today's highly stressed society. Nutrition is very much a 'Cinderella' as a branch of medical science, and this has various important and damaging effects.

First, it is an under-funded science, and thus attracts comparatively few researchers of excellence. This means that journalists and others often find themselves dependent on the extrapolation of foreign research when forming opinions about British nutritional needs. It is obviously harder to check facts and substantiate conclusions at a distance. Moreover, research into dietary effects on one population does not necessarily apply to another. Thus a theory develops in America about the effect of a dietary component on human health; scientists in Britain lack the resources to instigate matching research; the media get hold of part of the story (probably from a pressure group with an axe to grind) and publicize the issue as a serious threat to public health that is being ignored by the Department of Health. Reluctantly, the government commissions research, and eventually (two to four years on) proves the supposed risk to be non-existent. But the public has absorbed the media view of affairs, and a new folklore has been established.

Of course, the opposite can be true as well, and recent history has its examples of disregarded warnings, acted upon only after some cost to human health. The mistaken use of low-fat milk products for babies and young children is a good example. However, that is not – as the more extreme health activists would assert – an argument for more restrictive and centralized food and health regulation. It is a clear-cut case for more knowledge, more nutritional research and *more public information and education.*

The second effect of this neglect of nutrition as a serious life-science is that, regrettably, positions of influence in nutritional departments, on committees and in other organs of planning and legislation, at local and national levels, can become havens for people who are unqualified, or otherwise unsuited to hold them. This unsuitability can and does take the form of ignorance and/or vested interest. Much publicity has been devoted to the undue influence of industry on government advisory committees, but the position is no less potentially damaging to the public interest if people, whose personal views transcend their scientific objectivity (if indeed they possess any!), occupy the same positions of power.

Turning now to the media, we see a similar picture. Not because individual publications are anti-government or anti-corporate – this is plainly untrue. Some of the more virulent anti-establishment reporting is carried in newspapers whose proprietors are bastions of the establishment. The reason has more to do with a lack of detailed, or even superficial, scientific knowledge of nutrition.

Of course, specific scientific qualifications are not required to write good and interesting copy about a scientific subject if the original information is, in the main, accurate and objective, but a good journalist should ask an independent source to check the information. This is often not possible, because – to paraphrase Mae West – 'an independent source these days is hard to find'.

Nor can it be held that newspapers always pursue total objectivity. Accuracy and fairness sell few newspapers. The battle for circulation is a hard-fought ruthless struggle, in which truth is often sacrificed.

Industry could have done much more to present a better-informed and responsible story about food than it has. That it has chosen not to do so means that food producers are now paying a high price in loss of public sympathy and trust.

The stubborn silence of the processing sector has encouraged the distribution sector, especially the big high-street multiples, to seize the initiative, and present themselves as 'the consumer's friend', claiming to have eliminated harmful additives from their products, and assigning 'wholefood' benefits to their own-label produce. Yet, both the products and the expertise come from the hard-pressed food processors who manufacture own-label produce on the re-tailer's behalf.

This interesting shift of power away from the processing sector may have given the consumer a slightly louder voice. But the consumer's demands are still represented by a body whose chief interest is the consumer's pocket. Who, then, speaks for the consumer? Sadly, every individual involved would claim that distinction, yet none can claim truthfully to have carried out the duty consistently and well. A shift in values and attitudes is required on all sides, if we are to avoid a crisis of confidence which *will* lead to serious and long-term damage to public health, simply because the public will give up listening *to anybody*.

At the heart of any change must come a full-blooded commitment to serious public education, which starts in primary schools and finds its way up through secondary and further education, into the medical schools and, through local authorities, out to adult education establishments. The information and data upon which the teaching is based must be *sound and scientifically accurate* – rather than politically, ideologically or commercially motivated half-truths, which constitute the bulk of today's so-called educational material.

But where is this impeccable information going to come from, and who is to disseminate it? However much the vociferous anti-commercial gurus protest, industry must play a role in any honest attempt to impart high-grade nutritional knowledge to the public. The bulk of the best-qualified scientists work within industry, and it is unrealistic to expect any change in this situation in the foreseeable future. Talent will always go where it is best rewarded, and with a few notable exceptions, this favours the private sector. If industry wishes to regain its lost credibility, then it must fund independent nutritional research in our universities, and it *must be* independent.

The investment would pay off. Research into the dietary effects of foods and food ingredients on human health will produce important spin-off developments of commercial as well as scientific value. Nutrition will once again be seen as a subject worthy of postgraduate study by talented students, providing a steady stream of qualified people into all levels of academic as well as commercial life.

The media – if they are genuinely as concerned about public health as the fevered headlines often suggest – should help to improve the public's knowledge by investing regular space and airtime in informative and accurately researched articles, rather than in the attention-snatching scandals and sensations which now constitute their coverage of the subject. For once Fleet Street might try producing copy to inform as well as frighten. Who knows, the public might even read it!

It may seem far-fetched to suggest that the government divert public funds into both pure research and genuine and objective public education, at a time when the prevailing political philosophy seems to be more in the manner of Midas than Hippocrates. However, it would do well to reflect on the savings to the National Health Service budget (not to mention industry) that could be brought about by a fitter, better-nourished and more efficient population.

We do not hold out much hope, ourselves, that this solution will prevail. The positions held by the various factions are too entrenched, the old order too strong, to embrace change willingly. Once again, as has been the case so many times in the past, public health will be the loser, unless the public itself begins to take charge of its own case. We believe that substantial numbers of consumers are already resolved to do just that. This book is designed to be a first step in the process of understanding *the facts* about the food we are sold: what happens to it in processing, and what happens to us when we eat it.

The book's contributors have scrupulously drawn on the most accurate and respectable sources of information available. Our backgrounds reflect science, the media and industry, but we can honestly say we were unduly influenced by none of them in writing the book. We devised the idea, our publisher advanced the funds, and the British Nutrition Foundation gave us full and free access to its information and resources, imposing no editorial constraint from any quarter.

The purpose of the book is to give those interested in nutrition an appetite for further knowledge, based on an accurate understanding of the basic facts about our food. If as a result of reading it, you are motivated to inquire about, to challenge or to change any of the information you receive, or products you are sold, then we will have succeeded in our task.

2 Food Economics

Are the scales of food production balanced in favour of farmers, processors, retailers or consumers?

Barry D Ricketts

The study of food economics is, in many respects, the study of the development of a society. The growth and increasing sophistication of any community, region or nation (or for that matter, collection of nations such as the EEC) is dependent upon how quickly and successfully the bulk of the population can free themselves from the chores of food production, and concentrate on other wealth and power-creating activities.

In the case of Western Europe, there has been a migration of labour from agriculture into industry since the beginning of the Industrial Revolution. This was greatly accelerated in the years following the Second World War, as new territorial boundaries and allegiances gave birth to a common European market, designed both to prevent future strife and guarantee future food supplies – later to become the EEC.

However, other forces have been at work. The development of agricultural machinery and chemicals has greatly enhanced productivity per hectare and at the same time reduced the labour force on the farm. This has led to more mouths to feed in the towns as people turned to urbanized industry for employment. Inevitably, the tools of technology and science were then brought to bear on the food processing and distribution industry, to bring greater efficiency to the task of feeding the people.

As the balance of employment, productivity and resources has passed from agriculture to food processing, so a third phase in the cycle now gives emphasis not to the processor, but to the retailer, responsible for selling the products of the farmer and processor to the consumer.

In the UK, and to a greater or lesser extent throughout Europe, the food industry, as represented by the manufacturer or processor, has declined steadily in recent years as an employer, wealth producer and consumer. In proportion to other industries, the industry still remains vast – three times the size of the UK coal or steel industries, even excluding the farmers – but as a proportion of national expenditure, food spending inexorably shrinks as the economy grows. The economic reason for this is simple. Political and social constraints ensure that food production grows more slowly than in almost all other areas of industry. (In the early 1980s, food costs in the UK rose 5 per cent less than all other costs.) To the family, this means that it is more profitable to have family members earning than cooking. The catering industry has been quick to respond.

What do we mean by 'the food industry'? Certainly not the farmer alone, although many regard the agricultural sector as the epicentre of food supply. In fact this is far from the case. Today's farmer is merely one cog in a very complex and integrated machine. He supplies some of the raw materials in an extremely diverse national diet, but whereas, just a few years ago, the farm and its produce were in close proximity to the ultimate consumer, today they are as remote as a printed circuit board manufacturer is from a television viewer.

So varied are our dietary demands, in terms of the way in which we wish to purchase and consume our food, that the majority of the population have no contact with the farm at all – unless they discover the novelty of 'pick your own' fruit, or occasionally visit a farm shop. Those who purchase food as it was when it left the farm are a declining group. Increasingly the tendency is for retailers to provide more and more convenience – cleaned, cooked and packed foodstuffs, complete frozen meals, requiring only a few minutes or seconds in an oven or microwave.

Many city-based lifestyles have almost entirely eliminated food preparation from the home, and this is borne out by the rapid growth of take-away food emporia of almost every ethnic origin, restaurants to cater for all tastes, and a cornucopia of preserved foods of all types.

To arrive at this incredibly diverse degree of choice in food, a huge injection of technology from a wide variety of sciences and industries has taken place, and these inputs must be granted a place in our definition of the food industry. Many of the providers of these peripheral goods and services have had as large an impact on our diet as that most perfectly packaged meal, the boiled egg!

It is useful to think of the food industry as a linear and peripheral set of industrial systems. An example of a linear system would be the grouping of fishermen, fish wholesalers, refrigerated carriers, fish processors and/or packers, wet fish-shops (where they still exist) or supermarkets. Its associated peripheral industries would be the ice supply industry, the suppliers of ingredients and chemicals used in the processing, colouring, smoking and preservation of the fish, manufacturers of packaging materials and the manufacturers of the specialized machinery used in the processing of fish, from basic handling through to sophisticated preparation, cooking and quality-control systems.

These peripheral industries are important, for without them many of today's commodities and branded products could not exist. This is especially true in the case of frozen foods, which, combined with almost universal ownership of household refrigerators in the UK, have revolutionized eating habits.

Indeed, the eclipse of the agricultural sector as the key factor in the food industry is perhaps best illustrated by the fact that European agricultural prices have an impact on only 30 per cent of the total cost of our food. In common with all other industry, the most important cost determinants in food production, processing and retailing are labour and fuel. Notwithstanding this, price inflation in food is still lower than in nearly any other manufactured item. This comes about for two major reasons:

1. By and large, the industry is fairly efficient. It has to be. Slowly declining markets, rising costs, and popular and political resistance to the concept of inflation-linked prices mean that farmers, processors and others cannot afford to waste anything.

2. Difficulty in recouping the full cost of material and fuel-price increases from the market-place means that the industry has invested heavily in mechanized forms of production, reducing labour to a minimum. This makes the manufacturer very dependent on high-volume customers, i.e. the national supermarket chains.

2.1 Fish from sea to table

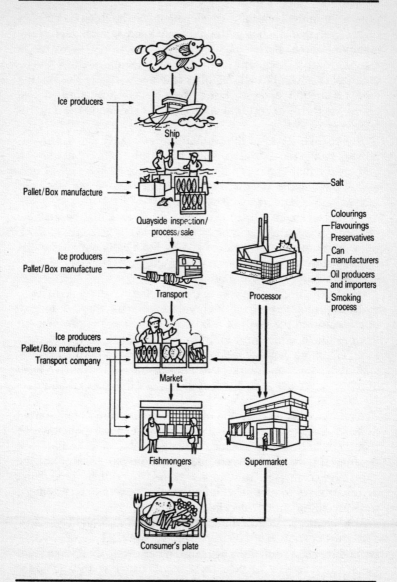

The retail revolution

One of the most important developments of the last two decades has been the emergence of the national chain supermarket as the dominant force in the food industry. Two store chains alone transact over 25 per cent of all grocery retailing in the UK. The purchasing power of such mighty combines is irresistible, and the food production and processing sector has succumbed almost entirely to the retail sector in deciding what goes on to the nation's table.

The changing role of the woman of the family, the deformalization of family meals, the readiness of consumers to try new foods, and the gradual spread of car ownership, have all played their part in popularizing the supermarket to the point where the small corner food shop has become a cult symbol.

The achievement of the food industry in extending the shelf-life of goods, and the chiller cabinet has enabled large stores to stock huge quantities of fresh foods at a considerable discount below the smaller store's prices. Consumers, quite understandably, have flocked to lower prices as moths to a flame.

By contributing in this way to the prosperity of the supermarket, manufacturers created the high-volume market they so desired, but also sowed the seeds of their own decline as the pre-eminent force in the food industry. Individual processors found themselves more and more dependent on very few customers for their profits. Gradually, the supermarkets demanded lower-priced, own-label products to sell alongside the manufacturers' brands, and stimulate further competition.

As the marketing expertise of the stores increased, they started to usurp – very successfully – the new product development which had hitherto been the province of the manufacturer. So intensive became the battle between manufacturers for space on the supermarket shelves, that many turned over their production almost entirely to own-label manufacture for very few customers, thus becoming entirely dependent on them.

Much of the success of these large retailers has been due to their size and location, and their perceptive exploitation of a socio-economic trend. But there was one other, even more important factor: they listened to their consumers. People were bombarded by products designed to meet their varying needs and lifestyles, and they liked it!

It would be an exaggeration to say that before the retailing revolution, food marketing was a technique used to promote the consumption of those products the farming and processing sectors could most easily produce, but it would not be entirely inaccurate. The existence of large, powerful buying groups, insistently reflecting public tastes and able to go elsewhere if the domestic industry did not respond, has focused minds wonderfully!

The dairy industry, for several years concerned about gradual declines in the high-fat liquid milk and butter markets, developed low-fat spreads and cheeses and made available skimmed and low fat milk. Manufacturers of meat products faced by increasing adverse publicity about sausages, developed low-fat versions. Low and no-additive versions of entire food ranges – jams, juices, tinned soups and fruits and pulses – were made available. Packaging was simplified to cut costs at one end of the range, and at the other, exotic foreign ingredients and menu items introduced foods seen before only on foreign holidays.

Perhaps the most significant factor from the consumer's point of view has been the increase in quality and value for money that the retailing revolution has engendered. It is not that food was of poor quality before the supermarkets began their campaign to dominate the food business; but the intense high-street competition led to a hitherto unprecedented concentration on perceived standards, which reached to every corner of the industry, and stretched as far back as the farmer.

The demise of farmer power

Farmers, beset on the one hand by quotas designed to reduce over-production and the surpluses to which they lead, and on the other by the impossibility of maintaining incomes at customary levels, are looking for diversification. Some will find new crops and products. A few will broaden their operations and become food processors as well as producers. Farmhouse-cheese manufacturers, intensive poultry units selling direct to the supermarket chains, and specialized market gardens supplying high-quality and specialized products direct, are examples of those who will survive. More will take large parts of their acreage out of food production altogether. Land taken out of agriculture cannot easily be returned to it. Reduced commodity production should, theoretically, reduce the cost of the Common Agricultural Policy (CAP), but in the long term, agricultural prices are bound to rise, as market forces replace the aberrations produced by farm price-support schemes and the over-production which resulted from them.

Higher raw-material prices, when they arrive, will demand even greater mechanization from the food processors in order to keep retail prices in check. This is almost bound to result in further rationalization of the processing industry. Production will be further concentrated into fewer hands, as weaker manufacturers go to the wall. Partnerships between farmers, processing companies and retailers are possible in order to guarantee the source of supply of vital food products to the stores.

At the other end of this scale, there is opportunity for the specialized producer and processor to exploit market niches for products which, by virtue of their enhanced quality or scarcity, will command a premium. It is unlikely that, for the UK consumer at least, basic food prices will match the inflation of other commodities. Although some constraint on production is likely to reduce the current level of surpluses, the very size and fecundity of the European farming resource, combined with the great political clout of the French and German farmers, will ensure that sufficient stocks of cheap grain, meat and dairy products are available to flood the British market, should our farmers ever become too demanding. It seems a great injustice that, by being resourceful and productive, and by observing the rules of the CAP, our farmers should have disadvantaged themselves as against their continental counterparts, but it is a political reality. The retailers have the power. They dictate the selling prices of our food, and if British farms and processors are unable to satisfy them, then others will.

Prospects for industry and the consumer

How have all the changes of recent years affected the standards, performance and basic values of the industry? Is today's consumer better or worse served by the food industry, and what can we expect in the immediate future?

That our food producers are more responsive now to consumer needs than ever before cannot be denied. Food today is cleaner, more convenient, there is greater variety, and food prices have increased less than most other basic commodities. Foods which meet the perceived values of 'healthiness' – low fat, high fibre, low sugar etc. – are increasingly available at economic prices to those who demand them, although these products have not been taken up by all sectors of society with equal speed and enthusiasm.

The industry has been accused of marketing too much fat, sugar and chemicals in its products for a variety of political and economic reasons. However, the facts demonstrate that as soon as a new dietary fashion emerges, so products appear to fuel the new trend. There have even been some examples of the industry *innovating* products based on advanced nutritional theories.

The purpose of industry is to make profit, not to bring about social change. It is unrealistic to expect it to be in advance of public opinion and demand. After all, the cost of installing processing equipment, developing new breeds of animals or finding new ingredients runs into many millions of pounds, and the investor has to be certain of a reasonable return.

Profitability in the food industry is traditionally lower than in other similarly capitalized enterprises. It has the virtue of commercial safety: people will always eat; there will always be a return. But if the food manufacturers are seen as slow in responding to perceived consumer needs, it is because they are cautious, not because they are indifferent to public health.

Certainly, the recent prominence of the retailing sector has significantly improved the responsiveness of the manufacturers. New markets are welcome to them, and the volume sales produced by the major multiples are hotly contested by all the firms involved. But there cannot be an ever-downwards spiral in prices without a gradual deterioration in quality. The store chains are aware of this, and the incidence of price wars shows some signs of decreasing.

Paradoxically, a cessation of price cutting for its own sake is in the consumer's longer-term interest. For unless the manufacturers are assured of a reasonable profit, they, like farmers, will cut their losses, and that will mean an end to the investment which guarantees tomorrow's new products and quality improvements. But are consumer concerns heeded by the industry, or are they mere indicators of a potential profit? Does the industry listen?

The majority of the consumer-representative groups seem to think that it does listen, that it is open and willing in its contact with the public. Of course, no industry is perfect, but the evidence from the food business, broad-based, diverse and multi-faceted as it is, reflects a consumer-aware industry. Virtually all major food companies have consumer-affairs or customer-relations departments employing qualified people, whose purpose is to deal with inquiries, complaints and requests from the public. The opinion held of the vast majority of food processors by the official watchdogs of consumer standards, the Ministry of Agriculture, Fisheries and Food (MAFF), and other regulatory agencies, is that they do their jobs well and maintain high standards of safety, hygiene and value.

It is true that there is a tendency for some industries to concentrate production in a few, large companies, which gradually take over smaller concerns. That is inevitable, as buying power becomes more concentrated and large customers need to deal with fewer, larger suppliers. But there is little evidence that this has tended to

2.2 Who owns what in the food industry - some examples

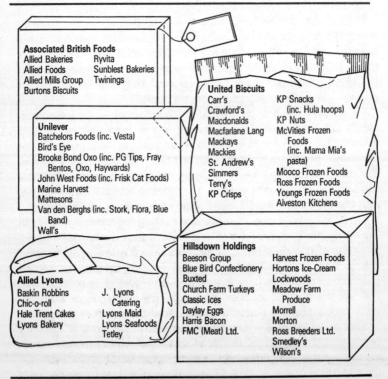

Associated British Foods
Allied Bakeries   Ryvita
Allied Foods   Sunblest Bakeries
Allied Mills Group   Twinings
Burtons Biscuits

United Biscuits
Carr's   KP Snacks
Crawford's   (inc. Hula hoops)
Macdonalds   KP Nuts
Macfarlane Lang   McVities Frozen
Mackays   Foods
Mackies   (inc. Mama Mia's
St. Andrew's   pasta)
Simmers   Mooco Frozen Foods
Terry's   Ross Frozen Foods
KP Crisps   Youngs Frozen Foods
                       Alveston Kitchens

Unilever
Batchelors Foods (inc. Vesta)
Bird's Eye
Brooke Bond Oxo (inc. PG Tips, Fray
  Bentos, Oxo, Haywards)
John West Foods (inc. Frisk Cat Foods)
Marine Harvest
Mattesons
Van den Berghs (inc. Stork, Flora, Blue
  Band)
Wall's

Hillsdown Holdings
Beeson Group   Harvest Frozen Foods
Blue Bird Confectionery Hortons Ice-Cream
Buxted   Lockwoods
Church Farm Turkeys   Meadow Farm
Classic Ices   Produce
Daylay Eggs   Morrell
Harris Bacon   Morton
FMC (Meat) Ltd.   Ross Breeders Ltd.
                       Smedley's
                       Wilson's

Allied Lyons
Baskin Robbins   J. Lyons
Chic-o-roll   Catering
Hale Trent Cakes   Lyons Maid
Lyons Bakery   Lyons Seafoods
                    Tetley

work against the consumer's interest. It seems to be more a function of nostalgia than logic to wish to protect the small business. Furthermore, the Monopolies and Mergers Commission exists to prevent concentrations of power against the public interest.

The final question must be whether the food industry and its products, as they stand today, tend to improve or worsen the health prospects of the majority of consumers? That is a deceptively simple question, for there is no such thing as a typical consumer, and although there are typical diets, they vary enormously in their effects. Dealing exclusively with economic rather than medical or scientific factors, the food industry has demonstrated conclusively on many occasions that it is capable of developing and marketing products which meet the requirements of responsible and well-qualified nutritionists and dieticians. That is their job.

Whether the community at large has taken full advantage of its food industry by practising sensible dietary habits is another question. Until our information and education systems are dedicated and organized towards consumer benefit, as the food industry has had to become, there will be room for dissent, suspicion and a failure to attain realizable goals in human welfare.

3   Food Politics

*Government, food industry, consumer groups and
the media constantly dispute food policy. Whom is
the consumer to believe?*

Barry D Ricketts

Politics is the undeclared additive in our food. It is inextricable and
all-pervading. Even at the level of the subsistence farmer, the political demands and customs of the outside world can intrude.
Drought-stricken nomadic farmers in Africa, forcibly moved by
their government to more fertile land, inspire international protests
to the United Nations in New York. By way of contrast, the Federal
Republic of Germany must heed the voices of its smallest farmers
when making European farming policy with other EEC partners,
for the collective power of this powerful minority can unseat
governments.

Food politics is by no means a straightforward subject. It operates
at many levels and involves a wide variety of vested interests. In
Europe, the parties and issues primarily represented in formal food
policy have been listed by D. R. Coleman in *Food and Health* (British
Nutrition Foundation, 1987):

Farmers and farm incomes
Regions dependent on agriculture and regional development
Food processors and distributors
Consumers, food expenditure, health and nutrition
Nutritionists and nutrition
Agricultural input supply industries
Environmentalists and the environment
Foreign farmers (ex EEC), food consumers and agro-industries
The balance of payments
The control of government expenditure

This is already a huge list when you take into account the individual
and group interests represented by, for intance, the food processors

and distributors, or as amorphous a group as consumers. Add to this the informal interests of the media, or the undeclared political agenda of some of the small sub-groups which exist within other major categories, and you have a recipe for confusion and mis-information unparalleled by almost any other subject.

The activities of both the media and the recent phenomenon of *ad hoc*, self-appointed groups claiming a nutrition or health interest are worthy of further examination, since they have been responsible for a considerable amount of public concern in recent years. They have covered a variety of dietary issues, some entirely relevant to public health, others owing more to political ideology than human nutrition.

These extracts from letters and responses written by Professor Conning, Director-General of the British Nutrition Foundation, in reply to issues raised in the media, give some indication of the topics in food deemed to be of political significance, and the mis-leading interpretation given to some of the subjects.

On fast foods

These arguments [against fast foods] use lack of balance to dramatize a point that would be seen instantly to be ludicrous if presented reasonably. No one in their right minds would live exclusively on sausages or ham-burgers or meat pies (or sweets or crisps) but the arguments are presented as if they would.

Comment, BNF, May 1987

On scientific integrity

The second [fallacy] is that scientists who have received financial support from industry or government are not to be trusted. Professional integrity can be judged most readily by quality of performance. In this respect the government's advisers have an impeccable record given that the nation's health has never been better.

Letter to *The Times*, March 1987

On food labelling

Governments and food suppliers have been too reticent [about nutritional content of foods] for fear that consumers may misinterpret the information and that health and commercial penalties may result. Well, a little know-ledge may be dangerous, but ignorance is worse.

Comment, BNF, June 1987

On the opportunist

The BNF is dedicated to helping the consumer understand the basis of good nutrition and abhors the anxiety and confusion created by the slogans of opportunist journalists and by misguided marketing strategies which together seek to cash in on the current interest in healthy eating.

Letter to The Listener, June 1987

On biased reporting

What I do denigrate is the influence of journalists and TV presenters who plug a given line that takes account only of certain facts (usually chosen for motives other than to inform) and MPs who cannot be bothered to make up their own minds, but merely adopt attitudes that are expedient vote-catchers. In these circumstances the public does not hear alternative arguments and thus cannot make an informed choice.

Letter to the British Medical Journal, October 1986

Activist strategies

There are undoubtedly two distinct trends in the more extreme and sensational types of food-related issues which confront us from time to time. There are those subjects which are promoted by serious health workers, motivated by genuine concern that the substance, syndrome or practice with which they are involved is being ignored, and should somehow jump the queue. They may well use political action to achieve their ends, and will most certainly use the media, and be little concerned about the effect on public anxiety. The second trend is the increasing use of so-called medical evidence or statistics to suggest that the current administration or policy is bad for people in general (or a deprived group in particular), and therefore the government or policy should be changed.

It is a common feature of both these techniques that they release information to the media *before* there is a general consensus of support for their hypothesis throughout the scientific and medical profession. Notwithstanding this lack of proof, the publicity accorded to the subject is so overwhelming, that by the time that radio, TV and the press have finished with the story, it has become a self-fulfilling prophecy.

It may, at first glance, seem odd that food should have become such a revolutionary subject in prosperous modern-day Western Europe. However, food has always been the strongest motivator to those who have sought the overthrow of governments. Hunger was the ultimate catalyst which fused the outrage of the French peasants and then the Russian proletariat into a force capable not only of overturning their government, but then creating a state which could effectively succeed it.

Hunger is not available as an argument to modern-day activists who seek similar far-reaching change. A substitute is required with similar fundamental appeal to rather better-nourished populations. What better than a conspiracy theory based on food? For example:

Farmers are landowners, and the party of government is their creature, basing its policy on what is good for the food producer, not what is good for the consumer.

Or:

There is a North v South divide in nutritional policy, whereby the deprived and largely anti-government North of the country receives a less-nourishing diet, and a lesser share of medical resources and general prosperity, than the more affluent and pro-government South.

It is tempting to take sides in this fascinating debate, but to do so prevents a proper understanding of the motivation and political bias of the many protagonists who profess an interest in the nation's food and health.

Conventional politics

First let us examine the status accorded to nutrition in the most recent election manifestos (1987) of the major political parties, in order to see how they perceive food as a vote-catcher.

The Conservatives claimed:

We have striven to bring commonsense to bear on the Common Agricultural Policy in the interest of taxpayers and consumers, while defending the interest of Britain's farmers.

Since 1979 productivity in agriculture in the United Kingdom has improved by well over 40%: we are more self-sufficient in food: our exports of agricultural products have increased by more than a quarter . . .

Under this Government, food prices have risen even less than prices generally.

We will continue to promote competitiveness and innovation in British farming and horticulture; . . . to encourage better marketing of agricultural and horticultural products and to ensure the consumer has as much information about the contents of food as is necessary to make sensible choices.

The Labour Party said:

To give Britain's producers the backing they need, the burden of agricultural support must be shifted from consumers . . . we will introduce new, long-term programmes for agriculture.

Labour will support the National Health Service and local government in providing more meals on wheels, . . .

The entitlement to free school meals and the restoration of nutritional standards are, like the strengthening of the school health service, commitments which are necessary to safeguard the physical and social well-being of growing children.

And the SDP promised:

The Alliance will promote a healthy farming industry. We must arrest the precipitous decline in farm incomes of recent years . . . adequate price and income support is required to enable necessary farming adjustments to be made . . .

The Alliance will work to reform the CAP. The policy has secured food supplies but has gone on unchecked to produce wasteful and hugely expensive surpluses.

We will seek a fairer share of milk quota for British producers . . . promoting healthy eating, tightening up food labelling and facing up to the problems presented by smoking and alcohol abuse.

When one of these political parties is elected, it has to give effect to these policies (where they exist) through legislation. This is the province of the civil service, which advises upon, and in some cases drafts new bills for Parliament to consider. It is also the responsibility of departments of state to administer the current food laws, and there is a vast and complex bureaucratic and scientific machine to carry out this responsibility.

The ministries with prime responsibility for food are the Ministry of Agriculture, Fisheries and Food (MAFF), the Department of Health and Social Security (DHSS) and, to a lesser extent, the Department of Trade and Industry (DTI). This latter department is principally concerned with the granting of development aid to help smaller businesses and encourage research.

These ministries are in contact on a regular, formal and informal basis with a number of other bodies who represent various groups during consultation, policy-making, research and enforcement. These groups are active both as lobbyists of, and collaborators with, the ministries. They include the National Farmers Union, the Food and Drink Federation, national consumer groups and many

3.1 Structure and relationships of MAFF food committees

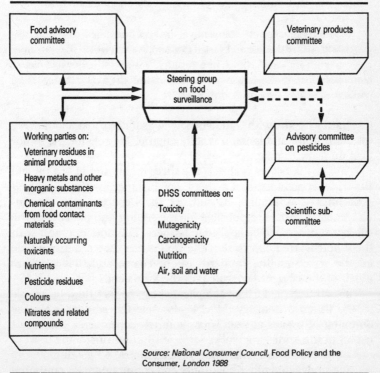

Food advisory committee

Veterinary products committee

Steering group on food surveillance

Working parties on:
Veterinary residues in animal products
Heavy metals and other inorganic substances
Chemical contaminants from food contact materials
Naturally occurring toxicants
Nutrients
Pesticide residues
Colours
Nitrates and related compounds

DHSS committees on:
Toxicity
Mutagenicity
Carcinogenicity
Nutrition
Air, soil and water

Advisory committee on pesticides

Scientific sub-committee

Source: National Consumer Council, Food Policy and the Consumer, *London 1988*

other organizations representing production, manufacture and processing, health and nutrition, health and safety and public information and education.

Two groups within MAFF are of particular significance in the formulation of public food policy: the Steering Group on Food Surveillance and the Food Advisory Committee. Consultation takes place within these groups with all those the ministry considers relevant to the subject at hand. Consumer committees are also mandatory in England, Scotland and Wales and, via a slightly different mechanism, in Northern Ireland.

This picture is much the same at the governmental level of most Western European and North American nations, and is very similar at the operating level of the European Communities Commission, which frames legislative recommendations for the member states of the EEC.

In Britain, MAFF, the leading ministry with regard to food-related matters, summarizes its own policy as follows:

... to foster an efficient, competitive, market-orientated food industry which will ensure the safe and varied food supply from which the consumer can make an informed choice of a healthy, varied and enjoyable diet at reasonable cost. It also endeavours to ensure that the food industry is in a position to exploit export opportunities.

It is hard to argue with that, embracing as it does, just about every relevant group and issue, a wholly appropriate role for the senior food ministry to take.

What few outsiders realize is the sheer immensity of MAFF and the wide scope of its total activity. For instance, as the competent department for farming, it, and not the Department of the Environment (DoE), is responsible for the setting and policing of the effluent standards to be applied to farmers. This does not meet with the wholehearted approval of the DoE, since they are responsible for the water-quality standards of our rivers, and that is where much of the effluent generated on the farms ends up!

This situation is further complicated by the fact that, in its role as the fisheries ministry, MAFF also sets the standards for the dumping of wastes at sea. There is much controversy about this aspect of the Ministry's work. Some authorities (including most of our other North Sea neighbours) claim that MAFF's dumping of sewage sludge and other pollutants and contaminants is poisoning the North Sea as a fishery. However, here at home we hear little of this; not surprising, since MAFF is also responsible for the quality standards of fish caught in the North Sea for consumption in the UK.

There may be no conflict at all between these various roles, given the way MAFF conducts its affairs, but it does seem an invitation to abuse at least, to allow one ministry to act as game-keeper, poacher, judge and jury in this way. Many critics – including the civil servants of other ministries – have in recent years called for a re-allocation of responsibilities between various ministries, in order to create greater public accountability.

Secrecy, conspiracy and complicity?

Confidence that the public interest is of prime concern for MAFF is not improved by the secrecy in which many of its committees and processes are clothed. The fact that a great number of the scientists serving the committees and working groups, which deliberate on such subjects as safety of ingredients and labelling, are drawn from industry is in itself unexceptional. It is quite appropriate that these highly experienced people, who know at first hand what is in our food, should make their expertise available in this way. But that their deliberations are sometimes covered by the Official Secrets Act, or shielded from public view under the guise of commercial secrecy, aggravates many already suspicious commentators and journalists. Some are convinced that there is a conspiracy between government and industry to deceive the public.

It is highly unlikely that conspiracy exists as a mode of official or industry behaviour. There are many examples of MAFF policies disadvantaging food producers and processors alike over the years, in a tireless effort to improve safety, quality and value for consumers. But the existence of such secrecy makes it very difficult to refute the claims of critics of government and industry, and gives rise to sensational charges from those who find MAFF's pace of change too slow for their radical turn of mind.

MAFF's very 'bigness' is not always a disadvantage. In fact, when it comes to dealing with serious and large-scale threats to the public health, MAFF is as good as any bureaucracy anywhere in the world. Its response to such threats as radioactive fall-out from the Chernobyl accident was immediate and thorough. Some have called it over-reaction, but it is impossible to please everybody! Such matters as national product withdrawal in suspected contamination incidents are managed with impressive efficiency. The minister's learned committees, which delve into food-related scientific matters important to public health, are thorough and all-embracing, giving favour to neither producer nor processor.

MAFF has always acquitted itself well in its scientific and practical help to the food producer. It has set up many schemes and processes which have produced tremendous improvements in standards of animal husbandry, soil and crop management, leading to agricultural standards which are the envy of the world. The consumer has been the nett beneficiary of all these initiatives, and the efficiency of the British farmer is acknowledged widely. But does the farmer wield an influence on the ministry which can lead to nutritional deprivation or damage among consumers?

It has been argued that the relentless race for ever more intensive production has produced the twin evils of huge surplus stocks, and excessive public consumption of so-called unhealthy foods – dairy products and red meat. This has been linked to a rising incidence of heart disease in Western Europe, and particularly, the United Kingdom (*see* Chapter 5).

Yet the truth does not support this assertion. In fact, the Common Agricultural Policy (CAP) has driven up the prices of dairy products and red meat in all EEC countries, leading to large-scale falls in consumption and a rise in the purchase of white meats and margarine (supposedly better for European hearts). That there are surpluses is certainly true, but that farming policy is unhealthy for European populations is quite insupportable.

Another criticism frequently levelled at MAFF is that the food industry has too great an influence on ministerial policy-making, leading to decisions which tend to favour the manufacturer rather than the consumer. Such criticism emanates, in the main, not from the representative consumer groups – many of whom play a part in the ministry's wider consultative processes – but from various pressure groups. A wide range of interests are represented by these activist bodies, many of them well motivated. The more responsible see their role as pointing out those tendencies within the food administration which may lead to dietary abuse on the part of the consumer. They tend to be purist and extreme in their arguments, and in their desire to promote healthy eating may suggest that the legislators wield the law-making pen more heavily in respect to some foods – for example, sugar, red meat, dairy products – than others.

However, MAFF does have a perfectly legitimate duty towards consumers, the medical profession *and* producers and processors, to ensure that proof of an adverse effect on human health actually exists, before action which may have far-reaching economic effects is taken. Those who criticize feel that it is better to err on the side of caution, and make a possible effect on human health a criterion. This difficult argument is at the heart of the political dilemma which constantly besets food legislators. To take an example outside the food industry, how many people would have avoided heart disease, cancer and other smoking-related diseases, had the strictures against tobacco been exercised before, rather than after, a long drawn-out period of research and resistance from the tobacco industry?

However, science, particularly food science, is not amenable to generalization. Nearly twenty years after the much-publicized 'killer cow' scandal turned rivalry between margarine and butter manufacturers into an international debate about the effects of dietary fat on coronary artery disease, we are still no closer to an answer to the central question: 'Does the amount or type of fat eaten by the individual have a predictable effect on that person's susceptibility to coronary artery disease?'

In the opinion of some, the fact that certain researchers and medical workers *believe* implicitly in a connection is enough. They interpret the reluctance of government to act in a determined way to reduce consumption of these foods as evidence of commercial interference. In fact, the ministerial response is infinitely more complex, consisting of a genuine concern that consumers be given information from which to make informed personal choices; that research from a wide and international field be accurately assessed; and finally, that the legitimate interests of an important and valuable national industry be protected from short-sighted, even mischievous interventions.

It is because the ministry's field of interest ranges so widely, that it is often accused of equivocation. However, it remains a good source of guidance and wholly accurate information to the concerned consumer about food. Publications such as *The Manual of Nutrition* and *The Composition of Foods*, available from HMSO, present a comprehensive survey of the constituents of our diet, and their known effects on our bodies. Specialized as these publications are, they are important as a countervailing influence to the misinformation which sadly characterizes much that is written in the popular press.

On the other hand, the DHSS has a more volatile political constituency, being primarily concerned with the public well-being, and has nurtured far more radical policies with regard to food and eating habits. This is a quite understandable state of affairs, given that the types of people employed, and objectives of the two ministries, vary so widely. In a field dedicated to the welfare of the people, it is unsurprising that DHSS has a higher percentage of individuals involved more politically in social issues, than MAFF.

Sadly, social zeal and scientific objectivity seldom make good bed-fellows, and many of the areas of mutual concern to the two ministries are characterized by a degree of friction. Whenever internal disarray becomes discernible to the media, it is pounced upon with delight and publicized. In recent years MAFF and DHSS have been accused of complicity in covering up scientific reports about a dietary divide between the social classes, of withdrawing school meals as a means of depressing the educational potential of poorer children, and a host of other seemingly Orwellian scandals.

Within DHSS is an infrastructure of concerned social workers whose priorities are the improvement of the lot of what they see as vulnerable groups. The scientists and administrators of MAFF are concerned to '. . . foster an efficient, competitive, market-orientated food industry which will ensure the safe and varied food supply from which the consumer can make an informed choice of a healthy, varied and enjoyable diet at reasonable cost . . .' Little wonder that there are differences of political opinion from time to time.

The confusing part, as far as the public is concerned, is the tendency of some journalists and activists to present this perfectly healthy clash of ideas – which probably tends to work in the public interest – as a battle between profit-motivated capitalists and public-spirited idealists, which almost certainly works *against* the public interest.

The million dollar question is, 'Does the food industry unduly influence departments of state?' The answer is that it probably tries to from time to time. It would be naïve to suppose that human nature and the pursuit of self-interest is uniquely suspended for the purpose of providing the nation's food. However, it would be equally silly to believe that our civil servants are not fully aware of the possibility of abuse and incapable of dealing skilfully with it. It is also silly to suggest that any major food industry or individual executive would seriously pursue a policy he or she *knew* to be detrimental to the public health. Consumers are only of interest to food producers and processors while they remain healthy, and of good appetite!

The question of influence remains and, undoubtedly, many try to influence the process of national food policy-making by lobbying Members of Parliament and civil servants. This is a time-honoured procedure, encouraged by government itself, in order to fully draw out all opposing opinions in an issue, before drafting legislation.

Lobbies and pressure groups

Lobbies and pressure groups exist right across the political spectrum. Some have been with us for years, in the form of clear-cut and established interests, such as the National Farmers Union, the Food and Drink Federation, the Retail Consortium and many others. Other organizations are more recent and reflect the development of consumerism as an organized force (*see* Table 3.1 below).

Often, the consumer-representative organizations are quite complex in the range of interests they cover and the strategies they pursue. It is perhaps inevitable that the area of consumer representation will be less well defined than that of, for instance, milk producers or potato growers. Their 'public' is a far more diffuse group, consisting of many levels of understanding, vulnerability, need, ethnic origin and prosperity. However, the existence of such a wide base requiring representation can provide a safe haven for those whose activities are directed against a particular industry or political party, rather than towards the improvement of national nutritional standards.

What makes this area of food politics all the more confusing is that 'false representation' is by no means the sole province of consumer representatives. There have been instances of commercial organizations covertly backing information campaigns which appeared to be independently compiled by concerned scientists, but eventually emerged as supportive of one or another product. Faced by such examples, it is little wonder that some political

Table 3.1   **Lobbies and pressure groups with an interest in food**

Animal Activists
British Independent Grocers' Association
Consumers' Association
Coronary Prevention Group
Farm and Food Society
Federation of Wholesale Distributors
Food and Drink Federation
Friends of the Earth
Health Visitors' Association
London Food Commission
Mother Earth
National Consumer Council
National Farmers Union
Public Health Alliance
Retail Consortium
Royal College of Physicians
Vegetarian Society

activists see the creation of fear about the food supply as a legitimate political tactic. From the public's point of view, this widespread tendency to use health fears to promote products or political points of view is highly undesirable, making it difficult for the consumer to differentiate between what is good for the family, and what is a commercial or political campaign.

Most of the organizations which lobby government are fairly self-evident, and their interests predictable. In the case of the producers, the National Farmers Union and marketing boards covering virtually all domestically produced food co-operate closely with government departments in the formation of policies which affect the quality, safety, labelling, and (for milk) pricing of their produce. The processors are similarly represented, at a general level by the umbrella organization the Food and Drink Federation, which has many standing committees and working parties covering the various sectors of the food industry. There also exist a number of discrete trade associations, which, although in many cases affiliated to the FDF, are separate from it. These organizations are legion and cover all the trades represented in the industry – milk, meat, fish, eggs, flour, fruit and vegetables, and cereals.

The trade associations have varying objectives, but they are mainly concerned with monitoring legislation that affects their members, and the protection and promotion of their market sector. They may provide information to the public about their products. Some of the most famous 'generic' advertising campaigns of all time were stimulated by trade associations and marketing boards. 'Drinka Pinta Milka Day' and 'Go To Work On An Egg' are good examples.

These promotional activities are, on the whole, harmless. They are very obvious, and have tended to follow nutritional trends fairly closely, although in some cases controversy has been generated by the use of advertising to try to reverse consumer trends motivated by health concern. To advertise cream at a time of national debate about obesity is to court criticism.

Less publicized is the work done by industry personnel in expert working parties with government. Although sometimes presented by critics of industry as 'sinister', this form of relationship is encouraged by all governments – regardless of political complexion – and aids the work of the civil service. It enables a particular expertise to be focused on complex topics and avoids the need for consultation with all firms represented in a given commercial sector. It also provides a mechanism for the presentation, at an early stage, of industry viewpoints on prospective legislation, without the need to 'lobby' MPs and mount delegations to various Whitehall departments. This does not mean that the industry does not lobby. On the contrary, if a political initiative seems to threaten an industry, the level of political activity can be as intense, and the use of media every bit as expert, as by any activist group.

By and large, the food industry's use of its relationship with government is useful and constructive, and the vast majority of items on the agenda are technical and non-controversial. But the fact remains that between industry and government will always stand the issue of how much you tell the public. Industry seems generally conditioned to be economical with information; civil servants have never been noted for their readiness to communicate freely with the public.

Enter the consumer groups

The role of the consumer group in improving the status of public nutritional knowledge cannot be overstated. The obstacles to be overcome by the genuine consumer representative, in transmitting knowledge, are formidable. At the level of party politics, food has never really emerged as an issue to rival, say, defence or nuclear power, or even sex-education in schools – this despite the fact that it is a universal subject, affecting all ages, ethnic groups and income levels. The subject has potential and far-reaching impact on education, health, economic policy, land utilization, the balance of payments and employment. Yet it scarcely merits a paragraph in party manifestos, and surfaces in parliamentary debate as superficial and piecemeal political carping. The last time a major debate took place on food in either House was in 1985.

Ministries are prepared to admit genuine consumer-representative organizations to their deliberations on some, but not all subjects. To an extent, it is up to the groups themselves to define the public interest as they see it, and work towards a system of representation and consultation which they regard as appropriate and open. This has been achieved in some Scandinavian and continental countries, but there are suspicions to be overcome before industry and legislators are ready to admit that the consumerist has a valuable role to perform in food policy-making. These suspicions are not helped if the groups themselves are overtly anti-government or anti-commercial in their initial approaches to any problem.

The National Consumer Council articulates well the dilemma facing serious consumerists in achieving a coherent policy-making role, and suggests some common-sense ground rules in this extract from *Food Policy and the Consumer* (NCC, May 1988):

Consumer organizations have to recognize that they will often be weak in relation to other pressures on the decision-making process for a variety of reasons, mainly that they have much more limited resources than the farming or industry lobbies. With restricted budgets and small executive staff, they have to co-ordinate grass roots opinion, obtain background information and expert opinion, and, on occasions, undertake their own research to formulate a 'consumer' view. Furthermore, they may be given fewer opportunities to consult. When put alongside the powerful, well-organized and by comparison, wealthy organizations which represent agriculture and manufacturing, it is hardly surprising that such a glaring imbalance exists. Arguably, mechanisms of consumer representation ought to be set up in order to redress this imbalance. But first of all, consumer organizations have to be clear about their own objectives and there is a need for consumer organizations to justify what they have to say by both demonstrating that they have a legitimate interest and that their views have some substance.

From the government's point of view, they are approached from all sides by people and organizations seeking to exert pressure and it cannot always be an easy task to distinguish between legitimate representation and self-interested lobbying. We are part of a political system which permits all forms of expression from the individual voice to the well-organized pressure campaign. Clearly there must be some way of identifying those consumer organizations which have a claim to be heard on an equal basis with representatives from the processors and from the industry.

For consumer organizations to justify a right of audience they should:

- have some kind of authoritative basis for what they are saying, either as a result of their own areas of research or on the basis of the views of those they seek to represent;
- express views which the government can reasonably be expected to need to know and take account of prior to making a policy decision;
- establish their own credibility for speaking on behalf of an interest group. It is difficult to define the precise nature of this credibility. It could be something that has come as a result of a proven track record for advancing submissions of quality and weight. Equally it could be a claim to speak on behalf of a large and representative membership;
- recognize their own duties in respect of being part of the consultative process. This means that they should be prepared to make responsible use of available data, and that they should make a considered and well-argued response.

It is criteria such as these which ought to determine whether or not any organization qualifies for the right to be consulted by government departments, to be invited to meetings and to expect that their views will influence the ultimate decision. Critics of the system suggest somewhat cynically that organizations have a much greater chance of being heard if their views are palatable and coincide with what officials want to hear. Undoubtedly the less dissension that is expressed, the easier it is for the officials to draft a policy which truly reflects the representations that are made. The process of consultation usually means that, when all the views are taken into account, we end up with a compromise which inevitably reflects political considerations and which may not be totally satisfactory for anyone. Consultation does not necessarily lead to acceptance of the views expressed.

As we have already seen, progress in areas such as food policy is rarely achieved overnight. It often takes years to achieve what might appear to be a very simple measure, based on sound consumer principles. As negotiations about food policy take place in Brussels as well as the UK, there is little hope of speeding-up the process. On the other hand, there is much that can be done to improve the effectiveness of the contribution of the consumer movement and to strengthen the influence they can hope to exert over such an important part of everyone's daily life. Food, after all, sustains us through life and takes up a significant part of every family's budget. Consumer representatives should expect to play a major role in ensuring its safety and wholesomeness and in receiving information about its composition and likely impact on their overall well-being.

The interface between consumer and industry has not been a totally depressing record. Of course, the consumer's ultimate sanction of non-purchase will always sway industry, but even this weapon will be less effective against, say, the liquid milk industry, where little local competition exists, than against food retailers, where the major names compete in every high street in the land.

This very factor has tended to produce a situation where the consumer movement has made greatest progress in its relationship with, and influence upon, the retail outlets. They in turn have brought pressure to bear on their suppliers, the manufacturing sector in this country and abroad. The result has been the appearance of many more products in the low- or no-additive range, whole-wheat bread, bakery and flour products, low-fat milk, sausages and spreads, and many other products in line with contemporary health fashions.

Some may doubt whether the availability of such products, in itself, improves the nutritional status of the individual consumer. But this is to evade the point, that consumer power has been applied, has had an effect, has caused a response and has enhanced consumer choice. Whether most consumers are able to exercise that choice in a way that will improve their nutritional prospects and those of their families is another and very contentious issue. The problem is that few authorities can agree on how good nutrition is to be implemented. There can be little doubt that this desirable goal is one that varies enormously between social groups and individuals. Nutritional status is different at various stages of the individual's life, and will also be affected by their general state of health.

What is required is a coalition of groups each representing a specific aspect of nutritional need – the elderly, the economically disadvantaged, ethnic minorities with special dietary needs, and not forgetting affluent groups, who can be equally at risk from poor nutrition – to provide a focus for sensible debate between industry (producers, processors and retailers), medical experts and those in charge of public policy. The various ministries would argue that that is exactly what the system of government represents with its expert committees and its widespread consultation procedures. If so, much better publicity should be given to the substance of their deliberations.

A forum might then emerge for the evaluation of nutritional theories, along with some consensus as to food-production priorities related to community needs, and – dare we hope – a realization that nutritional science has more worth as a tool to improve human health and quality of life, than as a short-term game of political football between the uninformed and the uncaring.

4 Basic Food Chemistry and Nutrition

All you really need to know about nutrients and what they do for you.

David M Conning

To enjoy both good food and a good diet, we need to know something about nutrition. What follows is the minimum information needed on food chemistry and nutrition to make some sense of the information thrown at us in newspapers, journals and on labels.

Food, nutrients and energy

The food we eat gives us nutrients and energy. Energy is what keeps our bodies working. Think of an engine. We know that it consumes fuel (petrol or diesel oil) but in fact it is the *energy* locked up in the fuel that drives the engine. Likewise, the energy locked up in food drives our bodies.

Nutrients are the basic materials that our bodies use for warmth, for growth and for repair. All our food is derived from plants and animals that have been alive. Simple chemicals, like salt, may be added to improve the taste but we do not need the extra amounts to survive. Nowadays many other chemicals are added to improve the colour, texture and keeping qualities of food but none has any nutrient value. They are used merely to keep the food palatable and attractive.

There are five groups of necessary nutrients: proteins, fats, carbohydrates, vitamins and minerals. Alcohol will also give energy but it is certainly not essential.

Proteins
Proteins are large molecules made up of chains of amino acids. There are over twenty different kinds of amino acids and several

4.1 How proteins are constructed

1. Amino acid chain

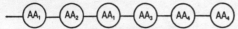

Amino acid chains. There are twenty different amino acids and they can be linked in any sequence so that, technically, there are hundreds of thousands of possible combinations.

The sequence is specific for any one protein and probably also determines how the chain is folded upon itself.

2. Protein

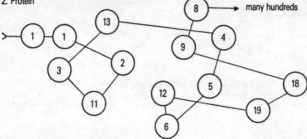

many hundreds

The way the chain is folded is very important because the function of many proteins is dependent on their shape.

3.

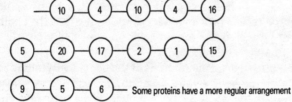

Some proteins have a more regular arrangement

Proteins with a more regular arrangement tend to form part of the body structure or have specialised activity like muscle or elastic tissues.

4.

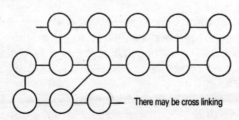

There may be cross linking

Cross linking adds to the rigidity and resilience of a protein, giving it a firmness and resistance to wear and tear.

4.1 (Cont)

---

5. Lipoprotein

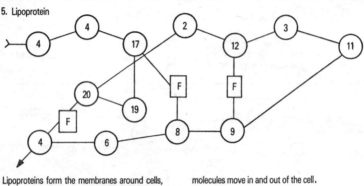

Lipoproteins form the membranes around cells, and have special functions in controlling the way molecules move in and out of the cell.
F = Fat

---

hundreds of different combinations are used for each protein. The different combinations and variable total mean that many thousands of different types of protein are possible. What is more, these chains of molecules are folded upon each other in very particular ways so that the type of protein also depends on the way the chains are arranged, as well as the amino acids present. Every protein is constructed to a very specific pattern.

Proteins are the structural materials of the body. Everything that goes to make up the body – skin, brain, lungs, heart, liver, bowel, muscle, even teeth – has some kind of protein as the basic material. Some proteins are combined with fat (lipid) to make lipoproteins, which have special properties for membranes and surface coverings. Others are arranged in very special patterns in muscles, which allows the muscle to contract when stimulated by a nerve. Yet others have special lubricating functions, say for joints, and there are specially toughened proteins to cover the joint surfaces. Almost all of the proteins used to construct the body are specialized in some way.

All these proteins are made within the body itself. When protein is eaten, it is broken down by digestive processes in the stomach and bowel to the component amino acids before they can be absorbed. No matter what the source of the protein is, it has to be reduced to the amino acids. These are then absorbed and used to reconstruct the particular proteins we need.

The best sources of protein are meat, eggs and dairy products – all animal proteins that have the full range of amino acids needed by humans. Vegetable proteins are not as good a source because not all plant proteins have the full range of amino acids. It is still possible to get the complete range from vegetables, however, by eating a wide variety of cereals, beans and seeds (pulses). Such a combination will provide all the requisite amino acids.

Fat

Fat (also called triglyceride) is a substance made from glycerol and fatty acids. There are three fatty acids to each molecule of glycerol. Fatty acids consist of chains of carbon atoms to which are attached hydrogen atoms and on the end of the chain is a special group, the acid group. The different types of fatty acids depend on the number of carbon atoms in the chain and on some special arrangements between certain 'links' in the chain. These in turn depend on whether a full complement of hydrogen atoms is present. If there is a full complement, the chain is simple and is called 'saturated' (i.e. it is saturated with hydrogen). If any of the hydrogen atoms is missing, the adjacent carbon atoms are termed 'unsaturated'. If there are several places where the hydrogen is missing, it is called 'polyunsaturated'. Such fatty acids break apart more easily.

As with protein, many different combinations are possible, so there are many different kinds of fatty acids. And as these can be arranged in many groups of three for attachment to glycerol, there are many different types of fat (triglyceride).

Fat is stored in adipose tissue and this is what we recognize as fat in, for example, meat. But in fact there is much more fat within the tissues because, in combinations with protein, fat is an extremely important material not only for structural purposes but for function. Many different activities in the living body are governed by the type of lipoprotein present, and because of the variable nature of both fat and protein there are many, many combinations each with its own function. Some fats are more specialized, having two fatty acids and one phosphoric acid, which may react with other compounds to produce what are called phospholipids.

Fat comes mainly from meat and dairy products and the vegetable oils extracted from beans, nuts and seeds. The fat in meat contains a mixture of saturated and polyunsaturated fatty acids, whereas vegetable oils in the main are monounsaturated (i.e. one link deficient in hydrogen) or polyunsaturated. Dairy products

4.2 Fats

1. Fatty acids

Saturated

$$-\overset{|}{\underset{|}{C}}-\overset{|}{\underset{|}{C}}-\overset{|}{\underset{|}{C}}-\overset{|}{\underset{|}{C}}-\overset{|}{\underset{|}{C}}\overset{O}{\underset{||}{C}}-OH \qquad \text{Acid group}$$

Monounsaturated

$$-\overset{|}{\underset{|}{C}}-C\diagdown_{C}-C-C-\overset{O}{\underset{||}{C}}-OH$$

Polyunsaturated

$$-\overset{|}{\underset{|}{C}}-C-C\diagup_{C}-C\diagup_{C}$$
$$\overset{|}{\underset{|}{C}}$$
$$\overset{|}{\underset{|}{C}}$$
$$C=O$$
$$OH$$

Fatty acids are chains of carbon atoms with an organic acid group on one end. If the link between any two atoms becomes unsaturated the chain is bent at this point. Several such points result in the chain bending back on itself.

2. Glycerol

$$\overset{}{\underset{}{C}}-OH$$
$$OH-\overset{|}{\underset{|}{C}}$$
$$C-OH$$

Glycerol is the simplest of the sugar-like molecules.

3. How fatty acids join to glycerol

$$C-OH \quad OH-\overset{O}{\underset{||}{C}}-C-C-C-C$$
$$OH-\overset{|}{\underset{|}{C}} \qquad \longrightarrow \text{water removed}$$
$$C-OH$$

Fatty acids are joined to glycerol by a process known as 'condensation' in which a molecule of water is removed. The resultant combination is known as an 'ester'.

4. Fat

$$C-O-\overset{O}{\underset{||}{C}}-C-C-C-\overset{|}{\underset{|}{C}}-$$
$$-C-C-C-O-\overset{|}{\underset{|}{C}}$$
$$\overset{||}{\underset{O}{}}$$
$$C-O-\overset{|}{\underset{||}{C}}-C-C-C-\overset{|}{\underset{|}{C}}-$$
$$O$$

| Glycerol | Fatty acids

Fats are fatty acid glycerol esters. The main form of fat has three fatty acids to one molecule of glycerol. This is a tri-ester, but is more commonly called a triglyceride.

5. Phospholipids

The fat involved with protein to make up cell membranes is usually a phospholipid in which phosphoric acid instead of a fatty acid is joined to one part of the glycerol molecule. This allows many other types of molecule to be tacked on giving a wide range of special functions.

These can be amino acids or sugars.

contain predominantly saturated fatty acids with some mono-unsaturated. Certain types of fish (herring, mackerel) are also rich in fat, much of which is of the unsaturated variety.

During digestion, fat (i.e. the glycerol with its fatty acids called triglyceride) is separated from any accompanying protein and absorbed. It may then be further broken down in the body and the component parts used to make whatever special fats are necessary.

Carbohydrates

Carbohydrates are a group of compounds made up of carbon and water and it is convenient to divide them into two main groups – sugars and starches – because that is how they occur in nature.

The sugars are further divided into single molecules (mono-saccharides) and double molecules (disaccharides). The single molecules are glucose, fructose and galactose. The double molecules are sucrose (glucose and fructose combined), lactose (glucose and galactose combined) and maltose (two molecules of glucose combined). There are many other varieties but these six are the only ones of importance in nutrition.

Starch is another chain-like molecule made up of strings of glucose molecules linked together. The chains may be very long and folded many times. The way these chains are arranged is very important to how starch behaves, especially in food preparation. As far as our bodies are concerned, starch is broken down, by digestive processes, to the component glucose molecules and

4.3 How carbohydrates are constructed

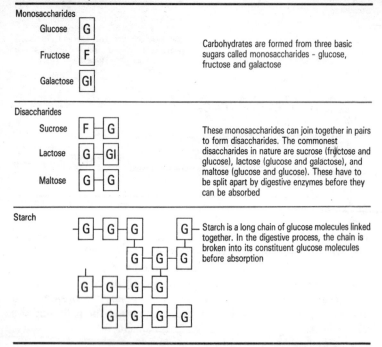

Monosaccharides

Glucose G

Fructose F

Galactose Gl

Carbohydrates are formed from three basic sugars called monosaccharides - glucose, fructose and galactose

Disaccharides

Sucrose F—G

Lactose G—Gl

Maltose G—G

These monosaccharides can join together in pairs to form disaccharides. The commonest disaccharides in nature are sucrose (fructose and glucose), lactose (glucose and galactose), and maltose (glucose and glucose). These have to be split apart by digestive enzymes before they can be absorbed

Starch

Starch is a long chain of glucose molecules linked together. In the digestive process, the chain is broken into its constituent glucose molecules before absorption

absorbed only as glucose. Similarly, the double molecules are broken down to their individual monosaccharides before absorption. So, in whatever form carbohydrate is eaten, the body only takes in glucose, fructose and galactose.

The main sources of carbohydrates are fruit (sucrose, glucose and fructose), milk (lactose) sugar-cane or sugar-beet (sucrose) and cereals (starch). Honey is sucrose that has been partially digested by the bee.

There is another kind of carbohydrate that has been hitting the headlines lately. This is dietary fibre, which used to be called roughage. It is derived from the structural tissues of plants or the husks of seeds (bran). It is another stringy material like starch, but this time made of different molecules, not glucose. Its essential characteristic is that it is not digested by the enzymes produced by the bowel and gives bulk to the waste material (faeces). As such, it prevents constipation and the complications that are associated with constipation. It also seems to have a dampening effect on the digestion of other foods, so that the absorption of nutrients proceeds more smoothly. As you would expect, we get most fibre from cereals, vegetables and fruit.

Vitamins

Vitamins are chemical compounds that are needed for many of the processes used by the body. They cannot be manufactured by the body and so have to be obtained from the diet. They act as catalysts and, as they are used slowly, only very small amounts are needed. Anyone eating a properly varied diet gets all the vitamins needed from food and does not need any supplements. Some foods are required by law to have vitamins added when they are used as a replacement for a common food that is a recognized source. For example, butter is a good source of vitamins A and D; therefore margarine, which many use as a butter substitute, is required to have vitamins A and D added. The main vitamins are as follows.

Vitamin A For healthy skin, resistance to disease and vision in dim light. Good sources are fish liver oil, liver, dairy produce, eggs and dark green and yellow vegetables.

Thiamin For the breakdown of sugars and starches. Found in wholegrain cereals, nuts, beans, meat and milk and yeast extracts (e.g. Marmite).

Riboflavin Also used by the body in the breakdown of nutrients. Found in dairy products, eggs, meat and yeast extracts.

Nicotinic acid Used in getting energy from food and needed for healthy skin. This vitamin can be synthesized by the body. The best dietary sources are liver and kidney, yeast extracts and wholemeal cereals.

Vitamin C (ascorbic acid) For healthy supporting tissues (the so-called connective tissues which hold the body together) and in the synthesis of some hormones. Found in citrus fruits, blackcurrants, salad vegetables (peppers, lettuce), cauliflower, spinach, potatoes and liver. This vitamin is particularly susceptible to loss during the cooking and storage of food.

Vitamin D Important for the absorption and use of calcium, this vitamin can be synthesized by the action of sunlight on the skin. Indeed, this is the main source because it occurs sparingly in the diet. It is found in oily fish, dairy products, margarine and eggs.

Of these vitamins A and D are soluble in fat and tend to occur in fatty foods. The others are soluble in water.

Minerals

Many minerals and metals are needed to keep the body healthy because they are used in many enzymes and in the proteins used to transport essential substances around the body. They are needed in exceedingly small amounts and usually a plentiful supply is available in any diet. Deficiencies occur only when there is excessive loss as, for example, of iron during bleeding, or failed supply as has occurred when patients are on prolonged intravenous feeding. The most important are:

Calcium Extremely important, not only for strong bones and teeth, but also for many other biological processes. It is present in abundance in many foods, particularly cheese, and there is a special mechanism for its absorption that depends on vitamin D. Its absorption is inhibited by phytic acid, a component of flour, and by dietary fibre, but these factors are of little significance in normal, varied diets.

Iodine Necessary for the proper functioning of the thyroid gland. The amount of iodine in food depends essentially on the iodine content of the soil and therefore varies. All seafood is a good source. Iodine is added to table salt in some countries where the soil may be deficient. This is not necessary in the UK.

Iron Essential for healthy blood and for the proper functioning of many enzymes. It is present in many foods, but that from animals is most readily absorbed. The absorption of iron from vegetables is improved by the presence of vitamin C.

Zinc Present in many enzymes and therefore essential for life. Although many effects of partial deficiency have been claimed, poor wound-healing is the only one substantiated. Good dietary sources are meat, wholegrain cereals, leafy vegetables and oysters.

Energy

Energy is measured either as kilocalories (the old Calories) or as joules (the European term). These are measures of heat or work.

$$1 \text{ kilocalorie} = 4.2 \text{ kilojoules (kJ)}$$
$$1000 \text{ kilojoules} = 1 \text{ megajoule (MJ)}$$

The body gets its energy from the major nutrients – protein, fat and carbohydrate – and from alcohol. As the nutrients are broken down, they provide not only the basic materials, such as amino acids, triglycerides and glucose, but also the energy that drives everything else. Alcohol is not a nutrient but, as the table below shows, it is a potent source of energy – and the reason why some people are overweight.

Table 4.1 **Nutrients and energy**

Protein	provides	4	kcals. per gram
Fat	„	9	„
Carbohydrate	„	4	„
Alcohol	„	7	„

The amount of energy a person needs each day depends on size and musculature, age, sex and how active they are. Labourers and sportsmen and -women need more than office workers; a muscular rugby player needs more than a paunchy businessman of the same weight. If more food energy is consumed than is used, the excess is stored as fat, a gain in weight that most of us experience in middle age when activity tends to decline but food consumption does not.

In general, a very active woman needs about 2500 kcals. (10.5 MJ) a day and an active man about 3000 kcals. (12.6 MJ). The rest probably do not need more than 2000 to 2500 kcals. (8.4 MJ) a day and many less than that.

Good nutrition

The essence of good nutrition is to eat as wide a variety of foods as possible but to keep the total intake of calories at a level that maintains an optimum weight. We need variety because *no one food* has all the nutrients the body needs. We need to guard against becoming overweight as that can lead to other problems such as high blood-pressure and arthritis (*see* Chapter 5). Although weight/height tables can give an indication of our 'ideal' weight, it is up to the individual to decide at which weight he or she feels most comfortable, and to arrange the diet to keep steady at that level.

Men have an additional problem, in that too much saturated fatty acid could be one of the contributing causes of coronary heart disease in susceptible individuals. It is generally agreed by most nutritionists that about one-third of our calories should come from

4.4 How many calories a day do we really need?

Light activity	Moderate activity	Heavy activity
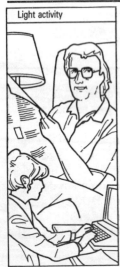		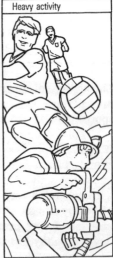
Most of the day spent sitting or standing e.g. office work. Little or no exercise e.g. rides to work, usually uses lift, watches TV.	Some time spent sitting but most of the day spent in activities that involve walking e.g. housework, postmen. Takes some exercise once or twice a week, e.g. sometimes walks to work.	Most of the day spent doing hard physical tasks - lifting, walking fast, e.g. athlete, builder. Takes some vigorous exercise every day.
Men　　2150-2500 kcal/day Women 1700-1900kcal/day	Men　　2750-2900 kcal/day Women 2150 kcal/day	Men　　2900-3350 kcal/day Women 2500 kcal/day

fat, just under half of which should be of the saturated kind. This means, for example, that a man who needs to take in, say, 2500 kcals. should consume about 42 grams (symbol g) of saturated fat and 56g of polyunsaturated fat each day. Most of us at present tend to eat a little more than that.

As fat is the nutrient with most kilocalories in it, eating too much of it encourages obesity. Regulating your intake of fat, therefore, will help keep weight down and reduce the risk of heart disease. Nevertheless, it is important to eat some fatty foods, especially saturated fat, because that is where the fat-soluble vitamins A and D are found in greatest abundance.

Protein ought to provide about 10 per cent of energy intake – say, 63 g a day for the 2500 kcal man. This leaves 55 per cent of calories from carbohydrates, say 15 per cent from sugars and 40 per cent from starch – 94 and 219 g per day, respectively. These figures allow about 18 g of alcohol a day for drinkers, that is about two units or a pint of beer on average. For teetotallers the daily amount of starch should be increased to 235 g. The chapter on practical nutrition will deal in detail with the ways these basic nutritional facts can be used in deciding upon and organizing your diet.

5 Diet-related Diseases

The facts about diet and health. Here is what we know and what we don't know. The rest is conjecture.

David M Conning

Food is a subject that everyone knows something about. We all eat, we know what we like and we all think we know what is good for us – or what our parents said was good for us!

The effects on our well-being of not eating enough, or of eating bad food, are quickly apparent. Not so obvious is the notion that what appears to be the right food for us might also cause health problems. Only relatively recently has it been realized that some of the foods we imagined were good might be the cause of those diseases expected in old age anyway – like heart disease and cancer. If this is true, is it not possible that other conditions such as mental illness, arthritis, or multiple sclerosis might also be due to faulty diets?

One would have thought that such important questions would give rise to long and painstaking investigations to find the answer. But nutrition, like all of the medical sciences, is a socially-conscious discipline, fearful of the damage that can be done by bad diet while waiting for the proof. As a consequence, recommendations for change are made when only a few like-minded nutritionists are convinced they are right. If these recommendations happen to coincide with the views of others with entirely different motivations (political or journalistic, for example) then a great deal of publicity is generated. It then becomes very difficult to complete research into that topic in a dispassionate and scientific manner. Other nutritionists, who are not yet convinced – and who resent being bulldozed for what they suspect are not scientifically sustainable reasons – react, generating conflict (itself the stuff of media hype), and a long row develops. The result is confusion and uncertainty in the minds of consumers who may well continue to eat what they have always enjoyed but now worry about it.

In this chapter, the evidence for and against a number of contemporary claims regarding diet and health will be examined to see if reasonable conclusions can be reached. First, however, we ought to consider what kind of evidence we need in order to prove that a particular item in the diet *causes* a particular disease.

Epidemiology and you

Human epidemiology is the study of a disease in a group of people. A major objective is to determine the cause. The 'group' may be a whole population, a section of a population, for example, of a particular age or sex, a community in a particular location or the workforce in a factory.

A *retrospective* study looks at people who have the disease or have died from it and tries to identify the causal factors to which they have been exposed. A *prospective* study starts with a group, identifies the factors to which they are exposed and, during a follow-up period – usually of a number of years – tries to relate the factors to the eventual development of disease. The latter kind of study often generates a more accurate impression of the factors involved. With the former approach, records and memories may be fallible.

The retrospective study is usually of a type known as a 'case control' study because actual cases of the disease (i.e. patients) are examined, whereas the prospective study is a 'cohort' study, where a group of people (the cohort) who have the factors to be tested is monitored for disease development. In each case a 'control' group is necessary. This is a group of people who match in every way the characteristics of the group under examination (the test group) except for the one (variable) being tested. This is not as easy to set up as it sounds, and might be particularly difficult for studies of the diet, where it is very unusual for large groups of people to have diets that do not overlap to some extent and have never done so. Some of the difficulties will become apparent as we consider the diseases.

Heart disease

The heart is a muscular pump that drives the blood round the body. It is active from before birth until death and never rests. Being muscle, it requires its own blood-supply to keep going and has its own blood vessels called the coronary arteries and veins. When a coronary artery becomes partially blocked, the heart muscle becomes short of the oxygen carried by the blood and cannot work properly. This results in a chest pain called angina pectoris. If a coronary artery is blocked completely, a sizeable part of the heart may die and the heart may stop beating altogether. This is a 'coronary heart attack' and can be instantly fatal, although modern medical treatment can sometimes keep people alive long enough for the heart to make a partial or even a complete recovery.

The blockage of coronary arteries is called coronary heart disease. In the UK about 30 per cent of men and 23 per cent of women who die annually, die of coronary heart disease. The peak age for this is 74 years and rising. The sad fact is that a large number of

5.1 Causes of death annually

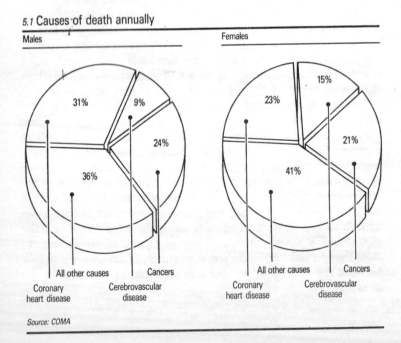

| Males | Females |

31%   9%   24%   36%

All other causes   Cancers
Coronary heart disease   Cerebrovascular disease

15%   23%   21%   41%

All other causes   Cancers
Coronary heart disease   Cerebrovascular disease

Source: COMA

5.2 The development of atherosclerosis

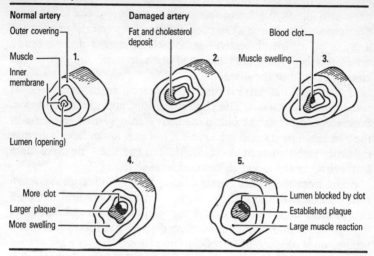

men die at a much earlier age – about 30,000 every year under the age of 65. No effort should be spared to prevent this tragic loss.

Blockage of the arteries (atherosclerosis or atheroma) is caused by a mixture of fat and cholesterol being deposited in the wall of the artery. This deposit occurs just beneath the internal lining of the artery, causing a swelling in the adjacent tissues. Often the lining membrane itself is damaged, resulting in a blood clot which seals the damaged surface. New membrane grows over the surface so that the blood clot is incorporated into the fatty deposit. The cavity of the artery is thus narrowed by what is now called an atheromatous plaque. As the disease progresses, and more fat and blood clots are deposited, so the artery becomes narrower, eventually blocking the artery completely. When the blood-supply is finally cut off, a coronary heart attack occurs.

Any artery in the body can be affected. If the vessels in the brain are involved, parts of the brain may die and the victim suffers a stroke. If it is the leg arteries, gangrene of the foot may occur. Kidney failure can result from the same condition in the kidney's arteries.

The precise cause of atherosclerosis is unknown. But we do know that it appears to start during adolescence and that almost everybody has it to some extent in old age. A great deal of work has gone into identifying factors common to sufferers, and it has been discovered that there is a direct association between the presence of a chemical called cholesterol in the blood stream and coronary artery disease. The higher the level of cholesterol, the greater the chance of getting the disease.

Cholesterol is a natural and vital component of tissues and is present in many foods. The cholesterol that appears in the blood, however, is synthesized within the body – that is, the cholesterol in the diet has only a small influence. What appears to have a greater influence is the amount of saturated fat in the diet – the more there is, the higher the blood cholesterol levels.

Apart from diet other habits that appear to influence coronary artery disease are smoking, alcohol consumption and exercise. People with high blood-pressure are also at greater risk. Smokers tend to suffer more heart disease, as do heavy drinkers (though a little alcohol tends to be beneficial) and those who take little or no exercise. These factors seem to influence the way cholesterol is moved around the body and the rate at which it is used up, rather than its production. People who are overweight are at greater risk too, possibly because they tend to have higher blood-pressure, as

5.3 Serum cholesterol and coronary heart disease

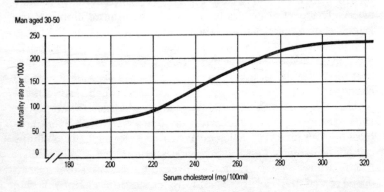

Man aged 30-50

Mortality rate per 1000

Serum cholesterol (mg/100ml)

This graph demonstrates that individual men with high levels of cholesterol in their blood run a greater risk of coronary heart disease.

It is also the basis for the advice that men should try to ensure their cholesterol levels do not rise beyond 220mg/100ml.

are those with diabetes. Heredity also plays its part. Some inherit a tendency to high levels of cholesterol in their blood, irrespective of the fat in their diet. It may be that this influence is at work to a varying degree in everyone.

There are thus several 'factors' linked with heart disease. To attempt to control for all of these in a study involving many people would make the study impossibly complicated and expensive. What is more, some of these factors (e.g. cigarette smoking) may not be affecting the coronary arteries directly but may be acting on one of the other factors, making the analysis even more complicated.

In these circumstances, it is very difficult for scientists who care about the truth to agree. Nevertheless, studies have been attempted which compare populations in different countries and groups within a population. Clearly, there are many lifestyle and cultural differences between countries and between individuals, making it difficult to find men in any one population who differ only in one particular characteristic. There is a measure of agreement, however, from such studies, that the level of cholesterol in the blood is influenced by the amount of saturated fatty acids in the diet, and that men with blood cholesterol levels above 250 mg per cent should try to eat less saturated fat.

What happens when that is done? Several studies have attempted to find out. In the definitive trial a large number of men were persuaded to take part in an experiment in which about half of them reduced their consumption of saturated fats, reduced or gave up smoking, and received treatment for high blood-pressure where necessary. Nearly 13,000 men aged 35 to 57 years took part and the study lasted around seven years. A preliminary study had predicted that deaths from coronary heart disease would be reduced by as much as 66 per cent in the younger men, though the trial itself was expected to bring about a reduction of 25 per cent.

After seven years, deaths from coronary heart disease in the test group had reduced by about 7 per cent, an effect that could have occurred by chance (i.e. not due to any changes in the diet etc.) and the overall death-rate was slightly increased, again a chance effect. In other words, a large and highly effective effort to persuade a large number of men to change their lifestyles to one thought to reduce the chances of a heart attack had no effect.

So what went wrong? One of the main problems according to the organizers was that fewer than expected in the control group died from the disease. As there is no explanation for this it has to be assumed that, whatever the cause, it also applied to the test group. All the so-called good effects, therefore, were due to some factor not being studied in the trial.

Usually, in these circumstances, scientists would abandon the hypothesis and try something new. In this case, particularly in the UK, attitudes have been unchanged, as though no trial had been conducted. Entrenched ideas and vested interests still pursue the diet/heart disease hypothesis.

Until we know better what *causes* heart disease, it is probably true that people will be better off if they reduce their fat intake, give up or cut down on smoking, seek treatment for high blood-pressure and take a little more exercise. They may not live longer as a consequence, but the chances are they will enjoy a better standard of health.

Cancer

Cancer, the most important of the human diseases as yet un-resolved, is the overgrowth of a group of body cells which even-tually invades the rest of the body. Nearly all cells can reproduce themselves when necessary, for example, during the repair of an injury. This cell division is well controlled by a mechanism not yet understood, so that when the repair is completed, the new growth stops. In cancer this control is lost and cell-division is unfettered.

What starts the cells dividing has been the subject of intense investigation for many decades. Environmental chemicals, hor-mones, viruses, radiation, asbestos and many other factors have been identified as causal factors. Recent attention has focused on the diet and, as so often in nutrition, many findings have been made – all conflicting!

In general, there is no good evidence incriminating any par-ticular nutrient or component of food as a *cause* of a particular type of cancer. But there is the possibility that several components interact to make it more likely that cancer could arise, whatever the cause may be.

Two things are reasonably certain. First, obese people get more cancer than people of normal weight. In women these tend to be cancers of the womb, gall-bladder, breast and ovary and in men, cancer of the large bowel and prostate. Animal studies have shown that more cancer results when the intake of energy from food exceeds the output over a lifetime, resulting in obesity. It has not been possible to confirm that a particular nutrient such as fat or protein is responsible, though there are advocates for both. It may be that an excess of energy itself is the cause. By what mechanism remains obscure.

Secondly, the consumption of alcohol is associated with a tendency to develop cancer of the oesophagus (gullet), though this is possibly due to chemicals present in alcoholic drinks rather than to alcohol itself. For drinkers who smoke, the chances of getting cancer are greater still. Cigarette smoking seems to be a habit that increases the chances of getting cancer and not just cancer of the lung. That is not to say that it is the smoking that causes the cancer. Rather, cigarette smoke seems to boost the cancerous process, either by preparing the ground for the actual cause, or by 'promoting' the cancerous process once it has begun. It is possible also that smoke diminishes the defences against the development of cancer. Whatever turns out to be the reason, there can be little doubt that the chances of avoiding cancer are improved by not smoking.

As far as other aspects of diet are concerned, nothing is certain and much of the evidence is conflicting. A number of food components are under investigation – fibre, vitamins and cholesterol.

Fibre   Dietary fibre, itself a mixture of several different types of carhohydrate, has been advocated as being protective against bowel cancer. This has not been supported by studies in Western communities where many other 'lifestyle' factors may be involved.

Vitamins   The multitude of chemical reactions that make up the process of living continuously produce compounds that could be hazardous if defence mechanisms did not exist. It is thought that vitamins (A, C and E in particular) are important for the proper functioning of such mechanisms, as is selenium, an essential trace element, vital for the proper functioning of several enzymes used in the same processes. These ideas are under intense investigation at present.

Cholesterol   The compound associated with coronary heart disease may also have a role in cancer. People with very low levels of cholesterol in the blood seem to be more susceptible to cancer than those with normal levels. It is not certain whether this is due to cancers not yet diagnosed or whether it is a true predisposition. Whatever is eventually proved to be the truth, it is unlikely to be a very serious factor in causing cancer.

All in all, it is unlikely that people on a normal, varied diet who keep within a reasonable weight range are going to influence their chances of getting cancer very much.

There is one other aspect of this topic that we should consider, however, and that is the effect of cooking – particularly of meat – by broiling or roasting. This has been shown to give rise to several chemicals that might cause cancer. Such chemicals have been shown positive in some screening tests and have induced cancers in experimental animals. It is not known if they can do so in humans, especially at the concentrations likely to be encountered. It remains a possibility, however, that many of the claims made for different nutrients are in fact due to changes induced by cooking.

Allergies

It has been known for a long time that people sometimes become 'sensitive' to certain foods. The word sensitive here has a special meaning, for it describes a particular type of effect on the 'immune' system of the individual. Everyone has an immune system. It is a means of defence against invading bacteria and viruses, whereby special proteins are produced that stick to the invading organisms, allowing them to be killed more easily by the defending cells that we also possess. Sometimes these special proteins themselves cause a reaction which we call an 'allergy'. Good examples are hay fever due to proteins provoked by pollen, and the gastro-enteritis which occurs as a result of eating shellfish or strawberries. Some people develop such allergies very easily, but for most of us they are uncommon.

Some sixty years ago it was suggested that many other symptoms such as a sense of fatigue, headaches (including migraine), anxiety and general malaise could also be the result of food allergy. The idea did not catch on at the time, essentially because there was never any supportive evidence of an immunological abnormality and the symptoms were so vague and variable. More recently, the idea has returned to fashion following the assertion that many children with behavioural disorders, particularly hyperactivity, were in fact 'sensitive' to certain foods or, more particularly, food additives and the claim that removing the offending substances from the diet effected a cure. This idea achieved such popularity that many parents imagined that every recalcitrant child was suffering from a food allergy and required special treatment. Sometimes, miraculous cures have been claimed through stringent manipulation of the diet.

It should be said straightaway that hyperactivity in a child is a very special and distressing condition that requires specialized knowledge to diagnose. A hyperactive child is not just a very naughty child and a naughty child is very rarely 'hyperactive'. Any parent who imagines their child is hyperactive must seek the advice of their doctor. It should also be stated that only in a very few cases where a food allergy has been claimed has an abnormality in the immune system been demonstrated. How then do we account for the improvement that many parents have claimed when they have modified the child's diet?

First, it has to be recognized that up to about five years of age, a child is meeting for the first time a whole range of foodstuffs not previously encountered for which a good deal of adaptation by the bowel and other bodily systems is necessary. This can result in vague abdominal pains, joint pains and itchy skin, which interfere with sleep and make a child irritable. At the same time, the brain is

---

5.4 The hyperactive child

Shows the following signs to an excessive extent particularly in the classroom. Teachers are good at recognising hyperactive children because such children are clearly very disturbed compared with normal children.

1. Restless, excitable, impulsive and fidgety.

2. Disturbs other children, interferes with their work, maybe aggressive towards them.

3. Inattentive, easily distracted, often fails to finish things started.

4. Appears frustrated, demands immediate attention, cries a good deal and has outbursts of explosive temper.

5. Frequent changes of mood.

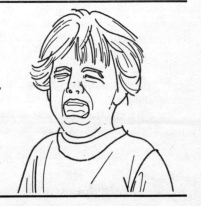

developing and behaviour patterns are being learned. The child needs a good deal of attention and sympathy during this lengthy period of adaptation, which for the child can be quite frightening. The child may achieve this attention by creating a disturbance, which then becomes a fixed reaction causing great distress to the parents.

One way of establishing a more constructive relationship between parent and child is to create a common cause in relation to the diet: something they can work on together. And there can be little doubt that for many parents this has been the key to a better understanding of the overall needs of the child, not just his or her dietary needs. Once this period of adaptation has passed, most children outgrow this reactive problem.

Occasionally parents overdo the treatment, putting the child on a diet containing too little energy – usually the result of misguided ideas about 'healthy eating'. The child then moves to the other extreme, becoming lethargic and failing to thrive properly, causing further anxiety for the parent. It cannot be stressed enough that if parents feel their child has a problem they should seek the advice of their medical practitioner – not least because there may indeed be a dietary problem that requires expert knowledge.

Diet and education

Another claim that has created considerable controversy is the notion that a child's educational attainment can be influenced by the diet. Although it is true that severe malnutrition can impair intellectual development, the main contention in developed countries is that some form of 'marginal malnutrition' exists due to over-dependence on processed foods. In the studies which are said to have demonstrated this, no attempts have been made to measure nutritional impairment, either of the foods or the subjects, and no study has used a change in diet alone to demonstrate the effect. In these circumstances, it is simply not possible to conclude that diet has any effect at all, and to claim otherwise creates needless anxiety.

The intellectual capacity of the population has been slowly increasing for many decades, so it seems very unlikely that current food-manufacturing practices are anything but beneficial, as far as nutrition is concerned. It does leave unresolved, however, the question of whether further nutritional improvement is possible, especially during the early years of childhood, and whether this could effect an improvement in educational standards.

Recent studies have suggested that boosting the intake of vitamin and mineral supplements improves performance in one aspect of an intelligence test, even in the absence of demonstrable nutritional deficiency. But much more work is needed before any worthwhile conclusions can be drawn. What can be said unequivocally is that properly-fed children do not need vitamin supplements.

Diet and body weight

Anorexia nervosa and bulimia

Anorexia means loss of appetite and occurs in association with several well-defined diseases. Anorexia nervosa, on the other hand, is an obsessional fear of being overweight that results in severe restriction of food intake with consequent emaciation. The subjects, usually adolescent girls, may be quite active, even athletic, but have an exaggerated impression of their own size. The cause is not known, but the patients frequently have unhappy family backgrounds and insecure personalities, and may suffer from depression. Occasionally the condition is associated with 'binge' eating where the subject consumes, usually in secret, enormous quantities of food and then undertakes self-induced vomiting or extensive and prolonged purging. This form of the condition is called bulimia.

Treatment is by prolonged and patient nursing, with psychiatric support where necessary, and may take many months. It is directed towards a gradual increase in energy consumption and the establishment of more stable and supportive family relationships. Most patients recover eventually, but some remain permanently thin. A few sufferers die, some from starvation or, more often, by their own hand.

Obesity

A person is described as 'overweight' if their weight is over one-tenth more than it should be according to height/weight tables, and as 'obese' if the weight is over one-fifth more (*see* Chapter 12). The excess weight must be due to fat and not to muscle and bone.

Thus many athletes (rugby footballers and weight-lifters) would appear overweight because of muscle development. The degree of fatness can be gauged by the thickness of the skin folds over the hip bones, beneath the shoulder blades, or at the back of the upper arm. These are best measured with special calipers; the total should be around one inch.

The cause of obesity is the consumption of more food energy than is used up by the bodily processes and by exercise. Although many overweight people claim not to over-eat, when in hospital they lose weight. Nevertheless, many overweight individuals do not eat excessively compared with people of normal weight. Either, therefore, they tend to be less active or they are more energy-efficient – that is, they extract more energy from a given weight of food. Whatever the reason, those who are overweight need to eat less and exercise more.

Overweight children tend to become overweight adults. Thus the lifestyle that results in obesity tends to be established at an early age. As there is a tendency for obesity to run in families, there may also be a genetic element.

Obesity is significant because it shortens life (*see* Figure 5.5) and because it is associated with a number of the diseases considered in this chapter (*see* Table 5.1). Being overweight is important because, although not a problem in itself, if unchecked it easily leads to obesity. It is much easier to retrain the appetite and develop better dietary habits at the overweight stage, than when obesity has become established.

5.5 Obese people die sooner

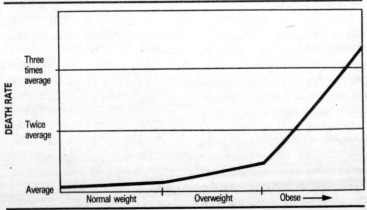

Table 5.1   **The perils of obesity**

Obese individuals have more	
Diabetes	Gout
High blood pressure	Arthritis
Liver disease	Hernias
Gall-bladder disease	Varicose veins
Lung problems	Skin problems

Diet and other diseases

High blood-pressure (Hypertension)

This is quite a common ailment among the middle-aged and the elderly, particularly men, which, if not treated, may lead to strokes or heart failure. It can be due to a wide variety of medical causes but there is one form, known as 'essential hypertension', which has, as yet, no known cause. The tendency to develop it is inherited, but much attention has been paid to the possibility that something in the lifestyle brings out a latent tendency. It is known, for example, that obese people develop the condition more readily than those of normal weight. Anxiety or stress may also provoke the disease.

For some time, it has been known that hypertension can be treated, at least partially, by reducing the intake of salt and this has led to a general assumption by some that excessive salt consumption may induce the condition. Indeed it is well recognized that some communities who consume very little salt tend to suffer much less from high blood-pressure, although it must be remembered that there are also other major differences in lifestyles. It is also true that Western communities tend to eat more salt than they need. The average consumption in the UK is 8–12 g per day whereas the basic need is for about 3–5 g.

Salt has always been valued for its food-preservation qualities and its role as a flavour enhancer, with the almost inevitable consequence that, as it became more freely available, the rate of consumption increased. Nevertheless, it seems probable that a liking for salt is an acquired taste and many can learn to enjoy much less salty food. Increasingly, food manufacturers are providing products with reduced salt content, which should be of particular value to sufferers from high blood-pressure. Salt substitutes, in which the sodium is replaced by potassium, are also available.

There is no clear-cut evidence that salt actually *causes* hypertension and there is very good evidence that too little salt is bad for the kidneys. But it would seem sensible that everyone should try to limit their intake to a maximum of 8 g a day. This would represent a reasonable compromise in that 3 g a day would mean no added salt, a diet that would be tasteless to many palates.

Other scientists have concluded that too little calcium or too little potassium in the diet contributes to the development of high blood-pressure. These findings have yet to be confirmed but, in any event, these substances are present in abundance in a varied diet. Increasing our intake may cause other hazards; for example, too much potassium interferes with kidney function.

For those who have a family tendency to high blood-pressure, the major factor is to keep body weight within normal weight/height limits.

Osteoporosis (soft bones)

There is a tendency for some women after the menopause to develop rarefaction (reduced density) of the bones, which may cause the bones to break more easily. Such bones appear less dense on X-ray because of the reduced content of calcium. This had led some nutritionists to suggest that it is lack of calcium that causes the disease, and to recommend that all middle-aged women should take extra calcium in their diets. The disease, however, is due as much to loss of the basic structure of the bones, which seems to be associated with the reduced production of ovarian hormones that occurs at and following the menopause. It is the loss of the bone structure that reduces the calcium content.

The best way to prevent osteoporosis is to ensure that the bones are strong and properly calcified *before* the menopause. This can be achieved by regular exercise and an adequate intake of calcium. The bones strengthen themselves in response to exercise. A properly balanced diet with adequate protein and dairy products (milk is the best source of calcium) will ensure this without the need for calcium supplements. Excess dietary calcium is a waste of money, as it is not absorbed.

It is now clear that hormonal replacement therapy (HRT) is an effective way of slowing down the rate of post-menopausal osteoporosis. Nowadays, the availability of this kind of treatment at low but effective dosage means that some of the fears of side-reactions are no longer valid. Prevention, however, is still better than treatment. Consult your doctor if you have any doubts.

Diabetes

This is a condition that can take two forms. In the first, glucose in the blood is not properly used by the body tissues because of a lack of insulin, a substance that is essential to allow the passage of glucose into the tissue cells. Insulin is produced by specialized cells in the pancreas. The only treatment for this form of the disease, in which the specialized cells are defective, is insulin injections. This form of diabetes tends to present itself during childhood.

There is another form of the disease which tends to occur in the middle-aged and elderly and is often associated with obesity. Here again there may be a lack of insulin, but more often there is resistance to its effects, many patients having an excess of insulin in the blood. This type of diabetes can often be controlled by attention to the diet. The amount of food eaten should not exceed that necessary to maintain normal body weight. Where the patient is obese, intake should be reduced until the excess weight is lost. The diet should be moderate in simple sugars, which tend to push up the blood glucose, and high in fibre, which tends to slow down the rate of absorption of glucose. Protein intake should be normal, but fat intake must be strictly limited since diabetics are more prone to heart disease than other people. Where dieting does not work, an oral hypoglycaemic medicine (such as tolbutamide) might be required.

One of the feared complications of insulin treatment is an overdose leading to hypoglycaemia, in which the levels of glucose in the blood are too low. This is recognized by feelings of weakness, hunger and, because of a reactive over-secretion of adrenaline, sweating, dizziness, palpitations and headache – all the symptoms associated with anxiety. This has led to the simple-minded notion that even ordinary people suffer from hypoglycaemia as a result of a reaction to too much sucrose in their diet. There is no truth in this crackpot idea.

Multiple Sclerosis (MS)

The cause of this distressing disease continues to baffle medical scientists. It is a disease of the central nervous system, characterized by loss of muscle control and paralysis which occurs in episodes interspersed with periods of remission in which complete, or almost complete, recovery may occur, only to be followed by a relapse at some future and usually unpredictable time.

It is not caused by dietary abnormality and is only included here because it has been found that the course of the disease can be modified (though not arrested) by diets supplemented by essential fatty acids. These are polyunsaturated fatty acids that cannot be synthesized in the body but are normally present in the diet in adequate amounts. They occur particularly in fish, meat and certain vegetable oils.

MS is a treacherous disease in that the periods of recovery often give rise to the hope that a particular treatment has been effective, only for the hope to be dashed by a further relapse. Supplementing the diet of MS sufferers with essential fatty acids has been found to cause some patients to experience less severe and shorter relapses, provided that the dietary treatment is started early enough. It is thought possible that the essential fatty acids are helping to repair the damage caused by the disease rather than curing the disease itself.

It is very unlikely that any diseases are *due* to dietary abnormalities, apart from the outright nutrient deficiencies such as occur in starvation and comparable conditions of deprivation. That is to say, a particular dietary aberration will not cause a disease. It seems very likely, however, that some diseases may be unmasked or made worse by bad diets, particularly diets that are unbalanced in respect of some nutrients. What this amounts to is that too much of any particular component is bad for the system and should be avoided. Moderation, these days, is considered boring but it remains the cornerstone of a good diet.

6 The Raw Materials of Food

Where it all begins and what is done to bring food from the field to the kitchen

David M Conning

Food processing is the conversion of raw materials into edible foods. In the narrowest sense, it is akin to the mixing and cooking of food that everyone does at home. In its widest sense, it also includes agricultural production on a global scale, the world-wide distribution of foodstuffs and their preservation, packaging and retailing. The food-processing industry now specifies very precisely the type and quality of agricultural products it needs, and organizes its production schedules to take advantage of the climatic and seasonal changes around the world. Items considered exotic only a short time ago are now available on supermarket shelves all year round. How all of this is managed is described in the chapters following, but for the moment let us consider why it is done and whether it is necessary.

In the old days (and not so long ago) people used to grow what they needed as food for themselves – most people in the world still live like this. The first requirement of any nation is enough agricultural produce to feed itself whether this is through the family plot, the farm, the collective or the massive combine. In a country whose economy is based on agriculture, large numbers of people are concerned solely with tilling and reaping, and tending animals. The success of such activity is dependent on the fertility of the soil, the availability of water and the control of pests, and is subject to seasonal vagaries. Life may be hard and uncertain. There is little scope for individuals to develop their lifestyles, unless they can extend their ownership of land and employ others to do the work. Furthermore, some way must be found to store food during the winter months when nothing grows, but stomachs still have to be filled. Food preservation has its origins in the resolution of this problem.

If or when a nation transforms to an industrial economy, increasing its wealth by the development of resources other than agriculture, there has to be an assurance that enough food will still be available, especially as such changes are often accompanied by an increase in population. The improvement in food supply is achieved either by increasing both the productivity of the farming community and the ability to store the produce, or by buying from countries that, by virtue of their over-production, have food to sell. Usually, increasing industrialization and increased agricultural productivity go hand-in-hand, but in some countries industrialization has developed to such an extent that the nation is no longer self-sufficient in food production. Advanced industrialization also brings increased numbers of city-dwellers with no opportunity for producing food for themselves. It has to be transported to them, often over long distances, and it has to be edible when it gets there.

As food science and technology have developed, many of these problems have been solved, and solved so successfully that in advanced countries food processing has extended into the home by the provision of 'ready to eat' food. Technology has enabled once-a-week shopping to become a common pattern, with the confidence that food can be kept for long periods without deterioration. These are the 'convenience foods' that have become such a part of modern life and have accompanied, and in part stimulated, a social revolution, particularly for women. Food preparation is no longer a chore but a choice. Anyone in the family is able to prepare meals, families eat out more, food is available at any hour of the day or night and, in general, people are better nourished than ever before.

There is a belief in some quarters that the 'revolution' has gone too far – that cooking should not be an art of the past, neither should our food be 'adulterated' with processing chemicals. Diminished taste and poorer quality are mourned and sometimes linked to health hazards such as arterial disease and cancer. The vested interests of large powerful food companies are seen as obstructive to the changes that might be necessary to ensure healthy eating.

Is there any truth in any of this? To answer, we must first understand what is done to our food and why. We will start with the processing of raw produce, without which we would not have much food at all.

Raw produce

Almost all foods grown require some processing to ensure they are edible or cookable or, as in the case of fruit, do not rot before they reach the consumer. In this sense, food processing is an ancient craft, though during the last fifty years it has undergone substantial industrial development.

Basically there are two sources of food: *animals* such as other mammals, poultry and fish; and *plants* such as vegetables (leafy plants), legumes (seeds from cereals, peas, beans and nuts), and fruit. In addition to producing meat, mammals give milk, which provides a range of dairy products, and poultry give eggs, while plants produce oils and sugars. All of these raw materials are processed to produce the foods that have become familiar to us. In this chapter, the various processes for converting raw materials into the basic ingredients used to make everyday meals will be considered.

Cereals

All grains have a similar structure consisting of a tough outer coat from which is derived the bran, a food store (the endosperm) containing starch, and an embryo or germ containing proteins, vitamins and a little fat (*see* Fig. 6.1 below).

Wheat

Processing is required to produce flour from the inner part (the endosperm) of the wheat grain. The grain is a tough structure that has to be broken apart during milling to get at the starchy interior. First the grain has to be dried, to prevent bacterial and mould growth, and then cleaned, to get rid of dirt, seeds and foreign matter. It then has to be 'conditioned', by being held in large containers for a day or two at the right temperature and humidity, to improve the moisture content throughout the grain, before milling.

In the milling process the grain is ground between rollers, and then sieved. Several grades of rollers and sieves are required to achieve the desired degree of flour 'extraction', that is, the proportion of the grain used to make the flour. The nutritional

6.1 A typical grain

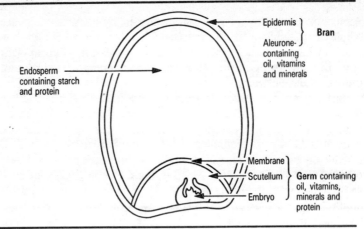

content of flour can be varied substantially by the extraction rates applied.

Because different nutritional components are concentrated in different parts of the grain (*see* Figure 6.1), considerable variations in types of flour can be achieved by blending the products of these grinding and sieving procedures. For example, the outer layers (containing bran) and the germ (containing oils, vitamins and minerals) are discarded for white flour but retained for wholemeal flour. The flour used for making brown bread retains part of the bran only, but not usually the germ. Thus wholemeal flour is 100 per cent extracted whereas white flour may only be about 70 per cent extracted. The texture of the bran in wholemeal or brown-bread flour may be coarse or fine.

The composition of flour is controlled by government regulations. The 'strength' of the flour is dictated by the amount and type of protein (gluten) present, which is in turn dependent on the strain of wheat, and determines whether the flour can be used for bread-making (high-protein) or for cakes and pastries (low-protein), especially if they are to be made on a large scale. Strong flour, used for making bread, has traditionally been produced from the 'hard' wheats grown in North America and Canada where long dry summers suit this type of grain. The kinds of wheat that thrive in the wetter climes of Europe are 'soft' and yield a flour with reduced protein content, more suitable for cakes and pastries.

In recent years, however, improved feedstocks have been developed through plant-breeding programmes designed to allow 'stronger' wheats to be grown in climates not usually suited to that type of plant. In the UK, for example, where the climate used to be suitable only for 'softer' wheats, it is now possible to grow the 'harder' (i.e. stronger) varieties that were previously imported. These developments may change the nutrient content only marginally, but will certainly increase availability and reduce the cost.

Rice

Although rice is similar in structure to wheat grain, the processing is simpler because it is not usually converted to flour but eaten whole. The process involves removing the outer 'hull', leaving 'brown rice'. Further milling removes the germ and the bran, and a final 'polishing' produces white rice. This milling is done with rough-faced spinning discs and polishing cones. As with wheat, the yield of good-quality rice is increased if the grain is 'conditioned' before milling by 'parboiling'. In this process, the rice is steeped in water for several days, steamed for a few minutes and finally dried in the sun. Surprisingly, the parboiling process actually increases the vitamin B_1 content by causing it to migrate from the outer shells into the endosperm.

Other cereals

Other cereals such as barley, oats, rye and maize (corn) are much less used as human foods in Western Europe though barley and oats are used for animal feedstuffs. The primary use of barley is as a source of maltose for browning and liquor distillation. This is because barley contains high levels of amylase, the enzyme that converts starch to maltose.

Oat is a grain that has little gluten, making it unsuitable for bread making. The bran is particularly adherent, and its removal involves steaming and rolling. There is some evidence that oats bran is particularly valuable as dietary fibre, but further work is needed for this to be established. The grain grows best in cool, wet climates and is well established in Northern Europe. The grain is high in fat content and a natural antioxidant, a chemical that prevents rancidity. A dusting of oat flour has sometimes been used to prevent fatty foods becoming rancid.

Rye grows well on poor soils. It is low in gluten and makes poor bread but is popular for crisp breads particularly in Scandinavia and Eastern Europe. Another characteristic of rye dough is its water-absorbing property, which some find useful to curb the appetite, as it swells up in the stomach. Rye is also used for alcohol production and as an animal feed.

Maize is the major cereal crop of North America though it is a relatively minor component of the American diet. Known in the USA as 'corn' it is used to produce cornflour, cornflakes and grits, depending on the type of processing employed. It is extensively used as an animal feedstuff and corn oil and corn starch find widespread applications in many industries.

Nutritional effects

The processes employed for grains do affect the nutrient content of the product compared with the native grain (*see* Table 6.1), but without them the product would not be palatable. Quite apart from the production of flours and meals, these products are supplemented nowadays to improve both nutrient content and palatability.

Table 6.1 Percentages of nutrient content of cereals before and after processing

Cereal		Moisture	Protein	Fat	Minerals	Fibre	Calories (per 100 g)
Wheat	Wholemeal	14.0	13.2	2.0	0.9	9.6	318
	Flour (white)	14.5	11.3	1.2	0.6	3.0	334
Rice	Brown	13.9	6.7	2.8	0.38	4.2	357
	White	11.7	6.5	1.0	0.34	2.4	361
Oats	Grain	10.0	12.2	4.3	1.1	8.0	319
	Rolled	10.1	12.0	6.8	1.8	7.0	361
Maize	Grain	10.8	10.0	4.3	1.5	1.7	348
	Meal	12.0	8.9	4.9	1.0	1.2	350

Meat, poultry and fish

The essential objectives of the processing of meat, poultry and fish are to optimize the quality of the product and to render it free of bacterial and fungal infections, and parasitic infestation.

Red meat

The quality of red meat depends on many factors, but the main considerations are the breeding and feeding of livestock to achieve the right balance between fat and lean meat at the time of slaughter; the skill of the butcher to ensure that the animal is in the optimum condition when killed, and that the meat is maintained at the proper state of hydration (water content) and temperature to minimize both bacterial growth and the release of those natural enzymes that cause deterioration.

The aim of these practices is, first, to keep the muscle as relaxed as possible before the animal is killed and rigor mortis sets in. This results in a more tender product. Hanging in a cool, dry place stretches the muscle (meat) and allows natural enzymes to break down muscle cells, producing a tastier product. The time required varies for different species and is, to some extent, limited by the amount and type of fat present in the muscle and by the inevitable microbial contamination. Nowadays, less time is allowed for these processes with a consequent reduction in flavour.

Tenderizing by means of enzymes (from pineapple juice, for example) is an old practice which used to be of limited value due to the difficulty of getting good penetration. Modern practice uses multi-needle injection so that the enzymes (branelin, papain and ficin derived from pineapple, papaya and figs, respectively) achieve uniform concentrations throughout the flesh. The mechanical process of the multi-needle injection on its own also has a tenderizing effect. Neither process is extensively practised now that the quality of raw meat has improved.

Similar devices are sometimes used to inject water into meats that are to be retailed in cooked form. This procedure facilitates slicing when the meat is subsequently cooled. (This process is discussed later in Chapter 9.)

Sausages

The great British 'banger', one of the delights of British cuisine, differs from its foreign counterparts in that its meat content is usually less. By regulation, the meat content is not less than 50 per cent for beef sausages (65 per cent for pork) but half of this can be fat. The remainder is cooked wheat flour (rusk) or bread mixed together with a 'binder' which may be egg, blood plasma, milk protein or soya protein. Very fine textured sausages (frankfurters) usually include emulsifiers, which may again be protein or trace amounts of a permitted additive. Commonly nitrite is used as a preservative.

Complaints about the reduced meat content of British sausages implied lower quality than continental counterparts, and products with a higher meat content are now available. Such sausages tend to be less succulent but can be 'improved' by the greater use of emulsifiers.

The salami type of sausage is generally made from raw ingredients, pickled in brine or smoked and air-dried. The initial process has a similarity with cheese-making in that bacteria are used to produce lactic acid. The meat ferments and it is heated, reducing the meat's water-holding capacity, so that it is more easily dried. Nitrite is also added during fermentation to help preservation and to produce the characteristic pink colour.

Originally the casings of sausages were made from the small intestine of the cow, sheep or pig (traditional haggis used the fore-stomach of the sheep) but nowadays almost all sausage casings are made from cellulose or collagen. Cellulose is extracted from cotton fibre or wood pulp and reconstituted in tubular form in an extruder. Collagen, a protein, is usually extracted from cow hides and reconstituted in a similar way.

Mechanically Recovered Meat (MRM)

Machines are now available that can strip the residual meat and fat from bones that have already been trimmed by hand. Some machines extract bone marrow at the same time. Both types incorporate sieves through which the meat is forced under pressure producing a paste with very little residual connective tissue (fibre and gristle). The resultant paste may be used to supplement the fillings of pies and sausages. MRM is particularly vulnerable to microbial contamination and should be rapidly frozen for storage, and rapidly thawed before use.

The use of such procedures, which are designed to reduce wastage, has been attacked on the grounds that a material of inferior quality is foisted on a gullible public to increase profitability for the

6.2 What's in a sausage?

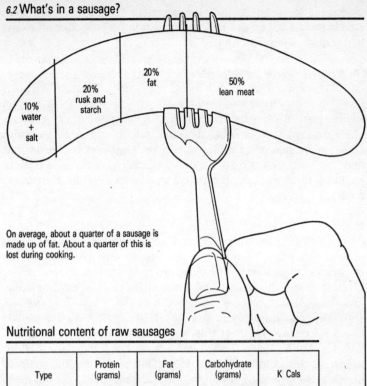

10% water + salt

20% rusk and starch

20% fat

50% lean meat

On average, about a quarter of a sausage is made up of fat. About a quarter of this is lost during cooking.

Nutritional content of raw sausages

Type	Protein (grams)	Fat (grams)	Carbohydrate (grams)	K Cals
Beef	10	24	12	300
Pork	11	32	10	367
Frankfurter	10	25	3	275
Salami	19	45	2	490
Saveloy	10	20	10	262

Each value is a weight equivalent to two large beef sausages food manufacturer. In fact, the objective is to use as much as possible of an expensive raw material and no reduction of nutritional quality occurs at all.

Mechanically Reformed Meat

Pieces of meat are 'massaged' together by very gentle tumbling in a drum in the presence of a salt solution. The effect is to express soluble protein from the meat and to increase the water content. The extracted protein coats the meat pieces, acting as a cement which sets on cooking, and results in a sliceable slab of meat that may be 'cast' in various shapes. A quicker process uses a more vigorous tumbling action but this results in substantial textural changes.

Poultry

Broiler chickens are specially bred for high meat yield and rapid growth. They are slaughtered at seven to ten weeks of age by stunning and bleeding. The birds are next immersed in water at 60 °C to loosen the feathers, which are then plucked mechanically, and the birds eviscerated, also mechanically. Birds to be sold as chilled are washed by spray and immersed in agitated water chilled to near freezing-point. At this stage there is some absorption of water which by law is limited to 5 per cent of the carcase weight. Where a bird is injected prior to chilling with polyphosphate to increase water retention and improve the succulence of the flesh, the 5 per cent limit does not apply, but the packed bird must be labelled as having been treated thus. Some carcases are deep-frozen (see Chapter 8). Turkeys and ducks are processed similarly, with minor changes because of carcase size. Birds from egg-producing flocks may be used to manufacture chicken meat products when their laying days are over.

Intensive farming

The urge to produce abundant supplies of relatively cheap produce has resulted in farming practices that minimize the labour-intensive nature of animal farming. This has meant keeping calves, steers, pigs and poultry in large sheds where the environment can be controlled and the incidence of disease limited. In these circumstances the animals are healthier and show better growth because their feed is better controlled and animal husbandry is more efficient. The animals are kept in confined conditions, however, and a few show signs that are thought to indicate stress.

Some believe that this is an unacceptable practice. They liken conditions to those of prisons and believe that the lives of the animals are degraded for the convenience of humans. What is more, they consider that, given the political manipulation of agricultural economics, with the resultant surplus production, such practices are unwarranted. Others are less concerned with the concept of animal rights, but believe that the intensive rearing of animals produces meat of reduced taste and eating quality. The force of the latter argument is less compelling because the aesthetic qualities of meat depend as much on processing expertise as on the husbandry. It is probably true, however, that in the urge to produce more, both factors are involved.

On balance, there is a general feeling, certainly in the UK, that the contemporary practices need to be modified, and research is under way to explore the efficacy of less-intensive rearing on the economics of meat production. Whatever the outcome, the cost to the consumer will increase. It may also be accompanied by improved quality and less guilt.

Fish

The quality of fish, the only wild animal now used extensively as food, depends almost entirely on low-temperature preservation. The development of processing ships to accompany fishing fleets has greatly improved the quality of fish reaching the consumer, as fish are best preserved if gutted immediately, 'glazed' (coated with ice) and frozen to at least $-5\,°C$ within an hour and then stored at -20 to $-30\,°C$. The fish are packed in permeable plastic film or paper. By law, transport temperatures must not exceed $-18\,°C$ as microbial activity in fish continues down to about $-10\,°C$. Other forms of preservation such as smoking may be used after the fish have been transported deep-frozen. They must be thawed rapidly before smoking.

Fish fingers are cut from compressed slabs of frozen fish. They may consist of one species (e.g. cod fingers) or several, or may be manufactured from minced fish. Occasionally polyphosphate is used to aid the retention of water, which facilitates processing. At present there is no legal minimum for fish content, though a product with less than 50 per cent fish (the rest being batter and bread) would not be a commercial proposition. It would seem preferable that the fish content should be displayed for the consumer's benefit.

Sugar

Sucrose, a compound of glucose and fructose, is obtained from sugar-cane from the tropics, or from sugar-beet which grows in temperate climates. Sugar-beet now accounts for about one-third of the world's production of sucrose.

Sugar-cane is cut into small pieces which are passed through a series of rollers under pressure to extract the juice. The raw juice is treated with lime to neutralize natural acids, boiled and allowed to clear (clarify) by setting. The juice is then concentrated by evaporation and the crystallized raw sugar separated from the residual 'molasses'. The raw sugar is refined by a series of processes involving washing, melting, suspension with calcium carbonate, filtration through granulated carbon and boiling under vacuum.

Brown sugar is the crystallized raw sugar separated from molasses before the final refining processes. It contains a number of other chemicals that give the colour and some flavour. It also contains 'invert' sugar, that is, some sucrose in which the glucose and fructose have become separated. This tends to increase the moisture content, making the sugar more sticky.

Golden syrup is the residual liquid derived from the final processes of refining white sugar. It consists largely of invert sugar and, usually before it is canned, some invert sugar synthesized from sucrose is added. Honey is sucrose about three-quarters of which has been inverted during the 'processing' of nectar by the honey bee. Sometimes, purified sugar is coloured with food dyes purely for decorative purposes. Such sugars are not used in commercial practice, such as the production of sweets.

The extraction of the juice from sugar-beet does not involve pressing but merely washing the beet pieces with hot water. The subsequent refining is broadly similar to the process used for cane sugar.

Fruit and vegetables

In relation to food processing, fruit and vegetables are special in that they continue to 'live' after harvesting. That is, they continue to absorb oxygen, give off carbon dioxide and generate heat in the presence of light. This not only affects storage conditions and the rate of ripening of the fruit, but also means that the adjustment of the atmosphere in the container during transport and subsequent storage plays an important role. The optimal concentrations of oxygen and carbon dioxide vary with different products. This atmospheric control method is almost always used with fruit but not with vegetables.

Generally, cool temperatures are needed to store fruit and vegetables though some tropical fruit are sensitive to cold and may actually need to be warmed. In recent years, with the advance of plant-breeding techniques and the ability to standardize the rates of growth and final size, quick freezing has become widely used for many fruits and vegetables.

The ripening of fruit can sometimes be accelerated when the atmosphere of the container has a small concentration of ethylene gas. This affects different fruits in different ways and has to be used with care, but is quite natural in the sense that many fruit generate their own ethylene gas as they ripen. This is why, for example, an apple helps to ripen avocados.

In picked fruit the commonest cause of spoilage is infection by moulds. This can usually be controlled by the avoidance of mechanical damage and by good hygiene, but some fruit, especially oranges, may be disinfected and coated with wax (which also helps prevent dehydration) or wrapped in paper impregnated with a fungicide.

The processing of raw vegetables is almost entirely devoted to preservation and depends on controlled humidity and low temperatures.

Pickling

This process was originally designed to preserve out-of-season vegetables. Now pickled food is recognized in its own right. Pickling is the preservation of cooked vegetables in acetic or lactic acid.

Pure acetic acid may be used. More commonly it is used in the form of vinegar, produced by the fermentation of sugars or starch beyond the alcohol stage to acid production (sour wine). Vinegar contains, therefore, in addition to acetic acid, other by-products of fermentation, most of which are unidentified.

Lactic acid is produced as a result of fermentation in what is known as the brining process. This is where cleaned and trimmed vegetables are immersed in a strong solution of salt which kills most of the bacteria and yeasts that abound on fresh vegetables. Some bacteria are resistant to salt, however, and it is these which – over the next three to six weeks – produce lactic acid by fermentation of the sugars and starches in the vegetables. After brining, some vegetables will also be conventionally pickled, but for some, such as olives and sauerkraut, brining is the sole process used.

Lactic acid is milder than acetic acid, and its preservative properties are not as good, so pasteurization (*see* page 82) may also be necessary. Sulphur dioxide, benzoic acid or sorbitol may also be added. We will deal with these processes in more detail later.

Organic farming
This involves a return to more traditional methods of land management. It arises from the belief that, in the end, the intensive use of chemicals to increase productivity reduces the agricultural quality of the soil and the aesthetic quality of the produce and carries with it inherent hazards to the consumer as a result of chemical residues.

True organic farming eschews the use of chemical fertilizers and pest-control agents. The consequences are reduced yield, greater loss through disease, substantial increases in the cost to the consumer – but, it is claimed, an increase in tastiness, and freedom from chemical adulteration. The method has gained some acceptance in affluent societies and an increasing number of small farms are converting to organic regimes.

Oils and fats

Oils are liquid and fats are solid. The difference is mainly due to the proportion of hydrogen to carbon in the fatty acids making up the oil or fat. The more hydrogen, the more 'solid' the product at room temperature. An oil can be made more solid by heating it with a nickel catalyst and bubbling in hydrogen under pressure. The degree of 'hydrogenation' which results depends on many factors including the type of oil, the temperature, the pressure and purity of the hydrogen, and the purity of the catalyst.

Vegetable oils

A variety of seeds, beans and fruits (e.g. sunflower, rape, maize, soya, olive, etc.) contain vegetable oils that can be extracted and purified, a process known as refining. The husks of the seeds or beans are removed and the kernels ground into a meal, or are flaked, before the oil is extracted, usually by a hydraulic press. Alternatively, the seeds or beans are heated to allow a solvent, such as trichloroethylene, to penetrate to help extraction. The solvent is removed later by evaporation.

The extracted material contains many components other than oil and has to be refined. After adding an alkali (caustic soda or lime) to neutralize natural acids it is again heated. Several stages of centrifuging and washing follow, all of which have to be carefully controlled to avoid damage to the oil itself. Finally, the oil is mixed with fuller's earth, heated and filtered under vacuum to decolourize it. Fuller's earth, a naturally occurring absorbent clay, has been used for centuries for the purpose of clarifying oils.

Butter

One of the oldest of food processes, butter-making has been subjected to advanced technical development in modern manufacture. What was traditionally a 'batch' process is now 'continuous'.

The making of butter first involves the separation of the cream from whole milk by centrifugation on spinning discs. The cream is then pasteurized (see page 82) and 'churned'. Churning is mechanized agitation that causes the fat globules in cream to coalesce into granules of butter, leaving the watery 'buttermilk' behind. Thus cream consisting of about 35 per cent fat and 65 per cent water is converted to butter consisting of 15 per cent water and 85 per cent fat.

After washing the butter, salt is usually added to enhance the flavour and to act as a preservative (inhibiting bacteria and moulds). The butter is then packed. Butter keeps better if it is packed immediately, thereby reducing the risk of contamination and exposure to atmospheric oxygen.

The quality of butter is to some extent governed by the size of the water droplets suspended in the fat. In the continuous process, pasteurized cream, at the correct temperature and acidity, is mechanically churned and the butter globules are forced through perforated plates with carefully calculated pore-sizes to produce uniform quality.

Margarine

Margarine was invented in 1869. At that time it consisted of a blend of clarified animal fat and cream, and was intended to be a close imitation of butter. Nowadays the main component is 'hydrogenated' vegetable oils, though animal oils or fats are used in a few blends.

The composition of margarine is controlled by law. In the UK, for example, it must not contain more than 16 per cent moisture or more than 10 per cent butter-fat. Low-fat spreads may differ, containing more water, but they cannot consequently be called margarine.

The manufacture of margarine is highly technical. Chemically, it consists of making a suspension of water in a blend of fats and oils (mainly hydrogenated in some blends). To add flavour the water component is often skimmed milk. The mixture (say 80 per cent oil, 20 per cent water) is agitated with an emulsifier to prevent the resultant mixtures from separating. There are many different emulsifiers that could be used, and these are described later. At the start of agitation the mixture is heated and then gradually cooled. As the fat begins to solidify, the agitation is reduced. The mixture is then rapidly cooled, mechanically kneaded and rolled to the required consistency, and packed. With modern machinery, this is a continuous process. The manufacturing system is very elaborate and all of the variable factors require close technical control.

Various additives may be used including salt, flavours and colours. Vitamins A and D must be incorporated by law to ensure that margarine, commonly used as a substitute for butter, is of comparable nutritional value.

Cheese

Making cheese from milk is another ancient food process, designed originally to preserve milk nutrients during the winter months when milk production declined. The process relies essentially on the precipitation of the protein component of milk by acid (curdling) and its subsequent modification by an enzyme called rennet (extracted from calves' stomachs). The acidification is brought about by bacteria converting the lactose in the milk to lactic acid.

The wide variety of cheeses depends on the variety of milk (from cow, goat, sheep, etc.), on whether the milk is whole or skimmed, on the different strains of bacteria used to produce the acid, and on various modifications of the process.

A 'starter' bacterial culture is added to warm milk and, when the required acid concentration is reached, rennet is added. The curdled protein together with trapped fat (curd) is separated from the residual liquid (whey), slightly heated and allowed to 'cure'. Salt is mixed in, the curd packed in cheesecloth and, depending on the type of cheese, subjected to pressure to remove residual water. After re-wrapping, the cheese is stored in a cool place for the final curing.

During curing or ripening, a process that may take several months, a number of chemical changes occur that are still not fully understood. Essentially, the protein and fats present are broken down to smaller molecules (peptides, amino acids and fatty acids). This results in a smoother consistency, closer texture and a variety of flavours and odours.

The large-scale manufacture of cheese follows the traditional process in all the essentials, but on a mechanized scale. Cheesecloth has been replaced by plastic or cellulose film.

Processed cheese is a pasteurized blend of natural hard cheeses with emulsifying salts (*see* Chapter 7) and skimmed milk or whey, to which colours, flavours or preservatives may be added. The resultant cheeses may be hard or soft depending on the residual water content and acidity. Sometimes in the manufacture of processed cheese the starting material is not natural cheese but a 'precheese' obtained by ultrafiltration of milk. Ultrafiltration is a process in which milk is forced through a synthetic membrane at increased pressure (about four times atmospheric pressure). The membrane allows water, some lactose and minerals through, but retains protein and fat in about the same proportions as curd. This can be fermented and treated with rennet as normal, the result being a soft processed cheese of bland taste. The advantage of the process is that some proteins, normally lost with the whey, are retained, thereby increasing the yield by about 20 per cent.

Cheese analogues are products made by blending milk protein with vegetable oils, emulsifiers, lactic acid and salt, followed by pasteurization. Different textures are possible by varying the proportions of protein and fat, and by modifying the acidity. Cheese analogues may be used for pizza toppings and in cheeseburgers. Different flavours are obtained by adding varying proportions of natural cheeses.

Colours, such as annatto or chlorophyll, may be added to cheese during manufacture. During the final curing, many cheeses have mould spores injected to induce changes in flavour, texture and colour (e.g. the veining in blue cheese). The mould most commonly used is penicillium rocheforti.

Milk

Milk consists of an emulsion of fat in a watery solution of protein, lactose, minerals and vitamins. The fat globules are maintained in suspension by a thin coating (membrane) of a special protein (lipoprotein). The detailed composition of milk differs according to the animal of origin and the time of the year, but the quality of the protein, the presence of vitamins and minerals, and the fat content make it a food of high nutritional value.

For this reason it is highly susceptible to microbial infection (bacteria also like good food) and much of the processing of raw milk is designed to counteract this susceptibility, while preserving the nutritional value and taste. As in buttermaking, the fat (cream) may be removed from milk by centrifugation. If this is taken virtually to completion, the residue is skimmed milk with a fat content reduced to 0.05 per cent (from 3.8 per cent). Semi-skimmed milk has a fat content of 1.5 to 2 per cent. Such treatments only affect the fat content.

To preserve milk as fit for human consumption several different methods of heat treatment are used depending on the degree of hygiene required. The main objective is to kill infection by tuberculosis, brucella and streptococcus. For this, 'pasteurization' is the method commonly used. For other purposes complete sterilization may be necessary.

Pasteurization The process involves raw milk being first heated and then cooled. In one method the milk is heated in a heat-exchanger and held in a stirred tank at 65 °C for 30 minutes and

Table 6.2 **The composition of margarine, butter, cheese and milk (per 100g)**

	Energy (kcals.)	Protein (g)	Fat (g)	Vitamins A (μg)	D (μg)	E (mg)	Calcium (mg)
Margarine	730.0	0.1	81.0	900.0	8.0	8.0	4.0
Butter	740.0	0.4	82.0	1220.0	0.8	2.0	15.0
Milk (whole)	65.0	3.3	3.8	57.0	0.03	0.1	120.0
Cheese (Cheddar)	406.0	26.0	34.0	515.0	0.3	0.8	800.0

then cooled. A heat-exchanger works on the same principle as a car radiator but with hot air or steam, rather than cool air, passing through it. In the 'flash' process, the milk is passed over heated plates, the flow being adjusted so that the required temperature of 72 °C is attained for 15 seconds. Both processes are commonly controlled automatically.

The conditions of pasteurization are such that there are no changes in the texture of the milk and very little change in the taste. The only nutritional change is a reduction in the amount of vitamin C, which is only present anyway in small amounts.

Apart from killing 'pathogens' (that is, bacteria capable of causing disease), pasteurization also kills a number of bacteria that cause spoilage. The keeping quality of the milk is improved but some organisms remain that will eventually sour the milk.

Sterilization Complete sterilization improves the keeping quality very considerably but the treatment adversely affects the milk's flavour. In the sterilizing process, filled bottles with secure tops are heated to 112 °C under pressure (in an autoclave) for 15 minutes. They are rapidly cooled to 80 °C and then allowed to cool slowly to room temperature. Recently plastic bottles have been developed which allow sterilization in a continuous process.

Ultra-high-temperature (*UHT*) Milk is heated to 132 °C for one second by passing it through a heat-exchanger. It is then packed under sterile conditions. Such milk will keep for six months or more at room temperature. There may be some change in palatability with this treatment but this is usually within acceptable limits and certainly much less than occurs in the sterilization process.

Despite the efficacy of heat treatments in killing bacteria, it is imperative that raw milk is handled under scrupulously hygienic conditions from milking to packing. All of the equipment, which should be glass or stainless steel, from milking-parlour to transporters to bottling plant, must be maintained in a high state of cleanliness and regularly sterilized with hot water or steam.

Homogenization To prevent cream rising to the top of the milk it is sometimes 'homogenized'. This process reduces the size of the fat globules in raw milk very substantially so that they remain in suspension. To do this the milk is forced under high pressure (140 kg/cm²) through perforated steel plates prior to pasteurization.

Evaporated milk The milk is processed to reduce its bulk – 87 per cent of which is water – and evaporated to a water content of about 75 per cent under vacuum at a temperature of about 50 °C. Small amounts of sodium citrate or phosphate or calcium chloride are added to improve the consistency, and the final product may be enriched with vitamin D. The milk is usually canned and sterilized. Skimmed or homogenized milk may be treated similarly.

When reconstituted, the milk is nutritionally unchanged. It is of value for infant feeding in the tropics, where supplies of fresh milk may not be available, though care will, of course, be required to ensure the sterility of water, bottles and teats. Evaporated milk has a characteristic taste and has become a dietary item in its own right for many people.

Condensed milk Evaporated and pasteurized milk has sucrose added to a final sugars' concentration of about 55 per cent (lactose plus sucrose). The sugar acts as a preservative (as, for example, in jam) and if the milk is packed in sterilized containers it does not require further treatment. It also keeps longer after opening.

Filled milk The butter-fat removed from skimmed milk is replaced by a vegetable oil such as corn oil. The milk is usually homogenized and supplemented with vitamins A and D to replace those lost with the cream. It is used quite extensively in catering.

Dried milk Milk in powdered form can be produced by a spray-drying technique in which pasteurized raw milk is pre-heated, condensed under vacuum to about 60 per cent water and then sprayed into a conical chamber through which dry air passes at a temperature of about 150 °C. The milk emerges as a fine white powder, which is then packed in airtight drums. The moisture content should not exceed 3 per cent. Some powders intended for the domestic market are 'agglomerated' to improve their solubility. This involves re-wetting the powder under carefully controlled conditions in a stream of air and steam before re-drying. This re-hydrates the lactose crystals.

The spray-drying process marginally affects the protein of milk in a way that produces 'antioxidant' properties which subsequently protect against rancidity. For products intended for industrial uses, lecithin, an emulsifier, is sometimes added to help reconstitution and prevent lumpiness.

Filled milk is also produced in spray-dried form and for this product antioxidants are permitted by law because vegetable oils are more prone to rancidity than milk fat. Products of this type form the basis of the so-called 'non-dairy creamers'.

Eggs

Eggs have high nutritional value because of their protein, fat, mineral and vitamin content. The protein (egg white) is very useful in food preparation, contributing highly desirable textural characteristics. Both of these properties tend to be lost as the egg ages, so the main objective in the processing of eggs is to preserve them as near fresh as possible.

During ageing, eggs lose carbon dioxide and moisture through the shell. Ageing can be delayed by storing in a humid atmosphere containing CO_2 (2.5 per cent). Other changes are due to the movement of water within the egg, making the yolk more fluid, and to chemical deterioration making the white watery. These changes render the egg susceptible to microbial infection, which can to some extent be counteracted by storage at 0 °C. Eggs may harbour salmonella infection derived from the hen, though this risk is greater in ducks' eggs. To avoid microbial contamination it is imperative that the producer maintains impeccable hygiene in his hen houses. Eggs should not be washed before storage as the water helps carry bacteria into the egg.

The widespread availability of fresh and graded eggs is due largely to intensive production using the battery system. In the UK, annual egg consumption exceeds 12 billion and it would not be possible to produce this number by any other method. Some people object to such methods and this has created a market for free-range eggs. However, the quality of free-range eggs cannot be guaranteed. It is important that those who prefer them get to know and use a regular supplier, that such eggs are not stored for long periods and that they are washed immediately before use.

Two egg products may be derived by further processing.

Frozen liquid egg Cool eggs from storage are washed in warm water and broken into a sterile bowl for inspection. This is done by hand and eye. The eggs are thoroughly mixed, filtered and pasteurized (63 °C for one minute). The mixture is then frozen in cans at a temperature of about -16 °C over about three days. In this frozen form it will keep for a long time. Sometimes the yolk and white are separated before freezing. If so, the yolk has to be treated with salt or sugar to prevent 'thickening'.

Dried egg Liquid egg, prepared as above, may be spray-dried after pasteurization. This process has to be carefully controlled to avoid the production of burnt flavours. To avoid deterioration and contamination, eggs to be dried must be as fresh as possible.

This then is the start of the story. Whether we like it or not, much food processing goes on before the food reaches the shops. If it did not, most foods would not get to the kitchen at all!

Most of the processes depend on heat and mechanical action and, when carried out on a large scale, take on the characteristics of an industry. The large scale does not reduce the need for careful handling; it increases it. And as the processes are complex and difficult to control, many operations are automatic and electronically operated.

All of this is a far cry from the myth of idyllic peasantry harvesting the fruits of their labour. But the pay-off has been food of a consistent quality and safety *for all*. Standardization has brought the benefit of consistently higher standards of hygiene and packing and controlled storage during distribution.

Whatever happens to food in subsequent processes, the basic processing of raw materials, as described here, is essential and will continue for the foreseeable future. In the next chapter, food preparation with some of the physics and chemistry involved, and some of the ways in which food preparation has been adapted to large-scale production, are discussed.

7 The Processes of Food Manufacture

The truth about industrial processes and how they compare with what happens in the kitchen

David M Conning

The processing of food involves the conversion of raw materials to edible products that collectively constitute meals, or are purchased to be incorporated into meals at home. Increasingly, the industry is involved in the production of complete meals and to many consumers this is what food processing is all about.

The food industry uses two basic processes, both of which mirror what is done in the home but on a larger scale. The first is the mixing of ingredients and the second is the application of heat or cooking. Each of these is a highly complex series of reactions that we normally take for granted and do not attempt to understand. But if you're in the business of manufacturing edible food by the tonne, these reactions have to be carefully controlled at all stages. Food manufacture is a highly industrialized process, which relies heavily on food science and technology.

Mixing

In all kinds of food processing, whether in the domestic kitchen or in the factory, mixing is a major activity. What is more, this mixing tends to be of dissimilar materials such as solids and water, solids and fats or oils, water and fat or, in whipping, air and fat or liquid or protein.

Technically, these mixtures are given different names. For example, a mixture of solids and liquids produces a 'suspension'; mixing dissimilar liquids produces 'emulsions'; and mixing air and liquids produces 'foams'. In food preparation it is quite common for two or three of these types of mixtures to occur together. Thus batter is an air–liquid–solid mixture, as is a soufflé. Often suspensions and emulsions are mixed as in sponge cakes, sometimes with foam folded in as with mousse.

The quality of cooking frequently depends on the efficiency of the mixing process, because this not only determines how well the ingredients are dispersed but also, and most importantly, it determines how small the individual particles are in the mixture. The smaller the particles (such as grains of flour or globules of fat), the greater the surface area and the more efficient and certain are the various changes that occur on heating (i.e. cooking) the mixture. This is because these changes happen more quickly and more completely – there is more 'room' in which they can work. Heat makes the starch in flour grains swell and form a gel (a kind of liquid jelly) that thickens the mixture and gives it 'body'. Heat also 'denatures' some proteins (i.e. sets them), but other proteins such as enzymes are 'activated' so that meat, for example, is softened and made more palatable. These reactions all occur more effectively in fine mixtures.

One way of achieving a fine mixture is to put a lot of mechanical energy into it through beating and whipping. There are, however,

7.1 Foams

Suspensions or emulsions with gas bubbles interspersed, e.g. aerated batter.

High magnification of a foam

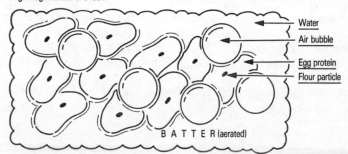

Water
Air bubble
Egg protein
Flour particle

B A T T E R (aerated)

On cooking, the starch in the flour forms a gel. This, together with the protein which denatures, converts the fluid mixture into a more rigid but still elastic structure.

Bread is similar, but the protein is gluten and the bubbles are carbon dioxide. In both batter and dough a little fat (from milk in batter and from the flour itself in dough) aid mixing.

certain chemicals that facilitate the process. These are called *emulsifiers* or *suspending agents*. They reduce the resistance between the phases (solid–liquid–water–fat etc.) so that less mechanical energy is needed to produce a finer mix. One of the best emulsifiers is lecithin (*see* page 92) which is found in egg yolks, hence the widespread use of egg yolk in cookery mixes. Some proteins such as albumin from egg white or casein from milk also act as emulsifiers. One can readily imagine that some emulsifiers are better for some mixtures than for others, and a great deal of effort has gone into finding suitable compounds for specific purposes.

Once a fine mix is achieved, there is a tendency for it to revert to the original state of two or three separate phases (air, liquid, solid). That is, there is a tendency for it to 'separate'. The finer the mix the less likely this is to happen, but some separation always occurs even with the best emulsifiers.

Such a tendency can be prevented by the use of *stabilizers*, that is, something to stabilize the emulsion or suspension or foam. The two commonest stabilizers are starch and egg white (egg white is virtually pure protein – albumin). The starch acts by forming a gel which greatly increases the viscosity of the suspending phase of the mixture – thickening it to make it more difficult for the suspended particles to coalesce. Protein acts in the same way when denatured by heat, whereupon it stiffens and holds the mix in a 'suspended' state. Protein is obviously very versatile as it can act as an emulsifier and then, on heating, as a stabilizer. Often, the art of cooking lies in the fine balance of getting all of these changes to occur at just the right time.

In the large-scale manufacture of foods, the proper control of the mixing and cooking processes is absolutely crucial, if the products are to have the consistency of form and quality that the consumer has come to expect. To this end, food science and technology have identified a number of different emulsifiers and stabilizers that work more efficiently in the widely differing situations that versatile food preparation presents.

Emulsifiers

Chemically, an emulsifier is a long molecule. One end is soluble in fat or oil and the other is soluble in water. For the fat-soluble end, fatty acids are commonly used. These are identical to the fatty acids which, in combination with glycerol, make up the natural fat of all living things. For the water-soluble ends, glycerol is commonly used or compounds derived from sorbitol. Sorbitol is a kind of sugar, similar in chemical structure to glucose and fructose (the commonest forms found in nature), but sufficiently different not to be used as a source of energy by living tissues.

Other emulsifers are simple salts made from sodium, potassium and calcium and the fatty acids. Yet others use the simpler organic acids such as acetic, citric or lactic acids (organic compounds are those found in living materials). The vast majority are made from naturally occurring compounds. Table 7.1 is a list of the emulsifiers permitted in Europe with their relevant E numbers. We will discuss E numbers later.

Table 7.1 **Emulsifiers permitted in Europe**

Lecithin (E322)
Polysorbates (E432–436)
Emulsifier YN (E442)
Na, K and Ca salts of fatty acids (E470)
Mono- and diglycerides (E471)
Acetic acid esters (E472a)
Citric acid esters (E472c)
Lactic acid esters (E472b)
Diacetyl tartaric acid esters (E472e)
Polyglycerol esters (E475)
Polyglycerol polyricinoleate (E476)
Propylene glycol esters (E477)
Polyglycerol esters of dimerized soya bean oil (E479)
Oxidatively polymerized soya bean oil
Sucrose esters (E473)
Sucro-glycerides (E474)
Na and Ca stearoyl-2-lactates (E481 and 482)
Sorbitan esters (E491–495)

Lecithin Probably the most widely used emulsifer, it is extracted from vegetable oils or seeds (usually soya or maize), or from egg yolk. It is used in fats, margarines, chocolate, toffee, bread, salad dressings and some instant drinks. It also finds uses in cosmetics, animal feeds and paints.

The following emulsifers, although related to chemicals that occur naturally, are manufactured. This ensures their ready availability at the standards of purity essential for use in foodstuffs.

Polysorbates Formed from the combination of sorbitol with a fatty acid and polyoxyethylene to increase the solubility in water. They are in widespread use as emulsifers but particularly in frozen products where they reduce the tendency of fat to crystallize. They also have extensive applications in cosmetics, pharmaceuticals and industry.

Emulsifier YN (ammonium phosphatides) Used essentially as a replacement for lecithin in the control of the viscosity of molten chocolate because, unlike natural lecithins, they impart no flavour to the product.

Fatty acid salts Used mainly as anti-caking agents (that is, to stop powders sticking together) but also in combination with other emulsifiers in a wide range of applications.

Mono- and di-glycerides Triglycerides are natural fats with three fatty acids to one molecule of glycerol. Where there are only one or two fatty acids, they form compounds (i.e. the mono- or di-glycerides) that are among the most widely used of all emulsifiers. They occur naturally as breakdown products of fats and are treated as natural products by biological systems. They are widely used in baking, confectionery, dairy products, margarines and potato or pasta products. They are also used in cosmetics, polishes, waxes and, somewhat surprisingly, in concrete.

Organic acid esters Widely used in combinations with other emulsifiers and in low-calorie foods where there may be a reduced fat content and increased water.

Polyglycerols Used most extensively in sponge and cake batters and ready-to-use mixes, they are good at preventing crystallization. Chemically, they are esters of polyglycerols and fatty acids and when eaten are digested into the fatty acids which are treated as such by the body, and the polyglycerols which are excreted unchanged.

Polymerized soya oil   In combination with mono- and di-glycerides, this is of particular value in margarine manufacture, especially margarines to be used for frying, where 'spattering' may be a problem. Spattering is due to the globules of water present and is reduced by reducing the size of the water globules.

Propylene glycol esters   Very widely used in the manufacture of baked goods, whipped desserts, icings and instant cake mixes.

Sorbitan esters   Esters of sorbitol and a variety of fatty acids are general-purpose emulsifers widely used in industry. Sucrose esters and sucro-glycerides should be classed with the sorbitans.

7.2 Emulsions and emulsifiers

An emulsion is a mixture of two immiscible liquids like oil and water. One is dispersed as tiny droplets (the discontinuous phase) throughout the other (the continuous phase).

Milk is an oil (fat) in water emulsion (i.e. water is the continuous phase).

Butter is a water in oil emulsion (fat is the continuous phase)

Emulsifiers are long molecules, one end of which is soluble in water and the other soluble in oil or fat.

Soluble in water   Soluble in fat

High magnification of emulsion - Water in oil

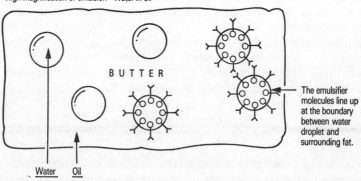

BUTTER

The emulsifier molecules line up at the boundary between water droplet and surrounding fat.

Water   Oil

Stearoyl lactates (sodium and calcium) Compounds formed from stearic and lactic acids and derived from natural compounds. They are separated during digestion and are treated by the body as the naturally occurring components. They are extensively used in the baking industry.

The wide range of emulsifiers described has come into existence because many of them are used in combination to achieve specific effects in specific applications. The development of many so-called convenience foods has depended to an extent on emulsifier expertise. As the currently available emulsifiers are, in the main, derived from natural products, they are assumed to be free from hazard. The majority have undergone extensive toxicity testing to confirm that this is so.

Stabilizers

The most commonly used stabilizers are starch and protein. Many different types of starch are used, all of them with different characteristics suitable for different applications. These characteristics relate to the viscosity of the gels, their rate of formation and dissolution, and the optimum temperature at which they are formed. Such variability may be an advantage but can also cause problems for a manufacturer trying to achieve consistency in his product.

One solution has been the development of 'modified starches' in which the chemical structure of the starch is altered by hydrolysis or oxidation. Such procedures result in cross-linking or better control of water-holding ability and allow considerable 'pre-tuning' of the particular activities required for particular applications. This produces a starch that will form a consistent gel under certain conditions and retain a clarity which is of value. Modified starches are now widely used as stabilizing and thickening agents, and the use of other agents has declined except for those with specialized applications. The other agents are listed in Table 7.2.

Gums Derived from plants or seeds, or the products of microbial activity, they have been used for centuries because of their ability to produce clear, tasteless gels. Being natural products, they tend to be variable in purity and consequently in performance. Nowadays

7.3 Suspensions and stabilisers

A mixture of a solid and a liquid in which the solid
is dispersed as tiny particles throughout the
liquid. Settling is usually prevented by a stabiliser
such as modified starch, protein, or gum.

High magnification of a suspension

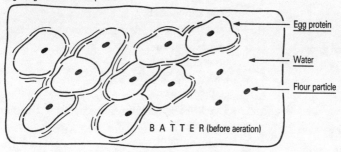

Egg protein

Water

Flour particle

B A T T E R (before aeration)

they are processed to a high standard of purity and some are also
synthesized. They are still used in confectionery and sauces,
although many of their functions are now more effectively achieved
with modified starches.

Seaweed extracts   Agar and carrageenan are polysaccharides (that
is, long chain-like molecules made up of different sugars) extracted
from seaweeds and have found wide use in food preparations, particularly ice-cream.

Pectins   Derived from plants they are of value because of their
ability to form gels under acid conditions and with high concentrations of sucrose present. Hence their use in jam, which was
originally devised as a means of preserving fruit.

Celluloses   Also from plants, they are used mainly in the manufacture of ice-cream (with carrageenan) and as stabilizers of foams.

Why are there so many emulsifiers and stabilizers and do we really
need them? There are two reasons why we have so many.
    First, food processing on a large scale is not subject to the loving
attention of the cook at every stage of the mixing process. It is not
possible when stirring several tonnes of a complicated mixture to
test by feel and sight the state of mixing achieved. Nevertheless, if it

Table 7.2 **Permitted stabilizers**

Proteins	Gelatin
Plant exudates	Gum arabic E414
	Gum ghatti
	Gum karaya 416
	Gum tragacanth E413
Seed gums	Locust bean gum E410
	Guar gum E412
	Psylum seed gum
	Quince seed gum
	Tamarind seed gum
Seaweed extracts	Agar E406
	Alginates E400–405
	Carrageenan E407
	Furcelleran
Pectins	Low methoxyl E440
	High methoxyl E440
Cellulose derivatives	Sodium carboxy methyl cellulose E446
	Microcrystalline cellulose E460(i)
	Methyl & methylethyl celluloses E461 & 465
	Hydroxypropyl & hydroxypropylmethyl celluloses E463 & E464
Microbial gums	Dextran
	Xanthan E415
	Beta 1-3 glucan

Note: Not all of these are permitted in the UK. This means mainly that they have not been included in the list of materials approved by the UK regulations. This exclusion does not indicate a problem with safety, but merely that no application for their inclusion has been made, an indication that UK manufacturers use satisfactory alternatives already on the list.

is not right, the final cooked product will not be right and nobody will want to eat it. In the course of time, therefore, food scientists have devised more compounds and mixtures of compounds, that, when used at the right concentration and with a given rate of stirring for precisely the right time, will produce a stabilized emulsion of precisely the right particle size and consistency, and which will repeatedly give a good finished product.

Secondly, although these new compounds may be readily used in established practice or lead to 'new' products, not all manufacturers can afford to experiment with the recipe of the products on which their livelihoods depend. Having found a combination of compounds that do the job and with which they have a lot of very satisfactory experience, they have no incentive to change. (Food manufacturers, like cooks, are by nature conservative.) This means that new compounds with more specialist applications may be added to the list but the old ones are retained. And so the list gets longer.

Is this likely to be dangerous? Not at all, for several very good reasons. First, any new compound for use in food has to be thoroughly tested (more of this later). Secondly, it has to be shown to do the job intended and that no other compound, already approved, will do the job well enough. Thirdly, introducing a new compound does not add to the total amount we eat – in fact it reduces the amount of *each one* we eat, in effect increasing the safety level.

Finally, if we were to return to using only traditional emulsifiers, there simply would not be enough to go round. Food would become more expensive and be reduced in variety. Consistency of quality and performance would deteriorate.

On the other hand, there can be little doubt that our chemical expertise has led to considerable standardization of food products, and to some standardization of tastes and textures. Whether this has gone too far is a matter of personal preference – a topic we shall turn to later.

Cooking

Human beings are the one species that eat only limited amounts of raw food. The use of heat to improve raw food – the cooking process – has probably played a highly significant role in the social development of modern man. Certainly, it has contributed substantially to the reduction of infection and parasitic disease.

The purposes of cooking are threefold:

1. to improve the digestibility and thereby the nourishing nature of food;
2. to destroy microbial contaminants and parasites, and to prevent spoilage by enzymes present in food;
3. to improve palatability by improving appearance, taste and texture.

The first two are more important (though only recognized relatively recently), but the third, and oldest, should not be underrated. Food that is not eaten has no nutritional value, and making food appetizing is a necessity not a luxury.

Heat is usually applied to food in one of three ways: as dry or radiant heat as in roasting, baking and grilling; as moist or conducted heat as in boiling, stewing or steaming; and by the use of very high temperatures as in frying. The application of heat has a number of quite profound chemical effects, many of which involve partial losses of some nutrients. These losses, however, are far outweighed by a general increase in the *availability* of most nutrients.

The effects of cooking on nutrients

Proteins

When protein is heated the arrangement of the chains becomes disorganized, i.e. they become 'denatured'. Although this usually means that the protein becomes less soluble in water, the unfolding of the chains tends to make the protein more easily digestible. This is particularly true of collagen which is 'hydrolysed' (that is, molecules of water are combined with the amino acids) thus rendering cooked meat less tough. In some cases a coagulative effect occurs, seen most clearly when egg white solidifies on cooking. Such a change is probably due to cross-linking between broken chain fragments.

Spoilage of food may be due to contaminating organisms, or to specialized proteins called enzymes present normally in the living material. The action of enzymes stops when they are denatured, so that heat treatment prevents spoilage from that source and cooked food remains palatable longer. It is for this reason that vegetables are 'blanched' or subjected to a quick burst of heating before deep freezing.

Carbohydrates

Starch   In its natural state, starch is difficult to digest. Heating in the presence of water causes the starch granules to burst and to 'gelatinize'. In the process, the starch molecules, which are long chains of sugar molecules (glucose), unfold and are much more readily digested. Cooking thus renders many vegetables, potatoes and cereals more palatable and nutritious. In some circumstances, the starch molecules break down to give molecules of glucose which may then become slightly 'caramelized' (see below). In this process the starch is said to be 'dextrinized' (dextrin is another name for small collections of glucose molecules), producing the golden-brown colour of chips and roast potatoes.

Sugars   When heated in slightly acid conditions – as occurs, for example, in the presence of fruit (jams and fruit pies) – sucrose is split into its two constituent sugars, glucose and fructose. This is known as 'inversion' and results in a sweeter mixture (fructose is sweeter than sucrose). It also results in a greater ability to retain moisture so that the food dries out less readily.

Higher temperatures lead to the formation of caramels from sugars. This change is valued for its attractive flavour and the brown colour it gives to the surface of prepared dishes. Another kind of 'browning' reaction occurs when sugars (or fats) react with the amino acids in proteins. These products are easily seen on the surface of roasted meat or 'honey roast' ham and are much prized for their flavour.

The individual cells that make up fruit and vegetables have special-ized carbohydrates in the walls consisting of long chains of sugar molecules, similar to starch chemically but different in format (the sugars are joined in a different way). These materials, the celluloses, tend to be difficult to eat and to digest. For some of them, cooking in the presence of water breaks the molecules apart, making them more palatable to most tastes and in some forms more easily digested.

Other types of chain-like molecules resist the effects of cooking and remain indigestible. These forms constitute the 'dietary fibre' that many nutritionists believe have for too long been ignored as an important part of the diet.

Fats

On heating, fats melt and facilitate the cooking process by transferring heat throughout raw foodstuffs. They may take part in browning reactions, creating attractive flavours, but are not themselves changed unless subjected to very high temperatures. When that happens they may decompose and give 'off flavours', some of which may be bitter. The brown products are different from those derived from sugars and starch.

Vitamins

Although heating generally improves the nutritional value of food, it may reduce the vitamin content. Some vitamins tend to be destroyed when heated in the presence of oxygen and water. This is particularly true of vitamin C (ascorbic acid), which is very readily broken down, but also occurs to a lesser extent with vitamins B_1, B_6, B_{12} and folic acid. Vitamins A and D (which are fat-soluble) are much more resistant to damage by heat.

In practice, the rate of destruction is only of significance for vitamin C, where some loss is inevitable. This can be minimized by using very fresh or deeply frozen vegetables, handling the vegetables gently, cooking briefly with minimum amounts of pre-heated water (too much water tends to wash the vitamins out) and serving quickly. Keeping food warm for prolonged periods removes virtually all the ascorbic acid. Happily, there are plenty of other sources of vitamin C (fresh fruit, fruit juices, etc.) and evidence of severe dietary deficiency of vitamin C (scurvy) has not been seen in this country for many decades.

The effect of cooking on micro-organisms

Normal baking, boiling or roasting procedures achieve temperatures that kill most micro-organisms and render food safe to eat. Yeasts and fungi are killed by moderate temperatures, but only the high temperatures achieved in canning and UHT treatments make foods virtually sterile. Mild heat can actually increase bacterial contamination.

Some bacterial strains produce 'spores', a form in which bacterial life is suspended for a time. Spores are much more resistant to destruction by heat but, given time and the right conditions, can 'vegetate' to reform the bacteria and re-infect the foodstuff.

Most organisms of this type merely cause spoilage but one, *Clostridium botulinum*, can produce a deadly toxin. The spores of *Clostridium botulinum* can only be heat-killed by the temperatures achieved in canning processes. However, because canned produce offers other conditions that would allow the spores to thrive (such as the absence of oxygen), the process requires extreme care and impeccable hygiene. The bacterium will not grow in acid conditions and for this reason food packed in cans is sometimes acidified when the food itself will not be affected. The growth of *botulinum* is also hindered by the presence of nitrites and nitrates (curing salts), hence their use as preservatives for certain meats and sausages.

Cooking and canning are so effective at controlling microorganisms that the main dangers arise from the later contamination of cooked foods. This is not to say that strict hygiene should not be observed with food preparation, but that the danger is greatest when the food has been cooked and is then kept at room temperature or re-warmed. Indeed, the danger may be increased further because contaminating organisms no longer have to compete with other species that have been killed by the cooking.

Despite the great improvements in food hygiene due to canning and modern forms of packaging, food poisoning is increasing, mainly as a result of careless hygiene in some domestic kitchens and catering establishments, and the slovenly behaviour of some people. On present experience, it can only be a matter of time before severe and lethal outbreaks occur. This risk increases if contemporary pressures to reduce the use of preservative chemicals succeed.

Obeying a few simple rules would do much to minimize the problem.

1. Keep working surfaces clean and wash the hands frequently.
2. Do not mix raw and cooked foods or use the same knife to cut them up.
3. Make sure your fridge works properly and store prepared foods above raw foods.

4. Make sure you use older items first.

5. Cooked foods that are to be kept should be cooled quickly but not in the fridge. Keep foods covered while they cool and until they are needed.

6. Make sure that any re-heating is done quickly and thoroughly.

7. Frozen foods, particularly meat and poultry, must be thoroughly cooked all through. This is best achieved by ensuring they are completely thawed before cooking starts.

Industrial cooking

The cooking of foods on an industrial scale is what most people understand by the term food processing or food manufacture. By now it will be appreciated that this is too restricted a definition, but it is probably this aspect that has the greatest impact on the consumer. In this section we shall deal with some of the processes that are used for commonly manufactured cooked foods.

Bread

Bread is essentially a delicate lattice of denatured wheat protein (gluten) throughout which gelatinized starch and carbon dioxide gas (CO_2) is dispersed. To create such a lattice, the gluten fibres have to be stretched and pulled to the right consistency, an effect achieved by mechanical manipulation and the creation of CO_2 bubbles. These bubbles result from the fermentation of sugars in the flour (a form of sugar called maltose) by yeast. The maltose itself results from enzymes present in the flour acting on the starch, an effect initiated by water.

The flavour of bread is also generated by other products of fermentation such as alcohols and organic acids, by the caramels and browning reaction products that occur in the crust, and by added salt.

Thus the essential ingredients of bread are flour, salt, water and yeast. Classically the process involves kneading to stretch the gluten fibres, and allowing time for fermentation to occur. Industry has found ways of speeding up this process. These include:

1. More powerful yeasts together with a mixture of yeast nutrients that reduce the necessary fermentation time to minutes rather than hours. The function of the yeast in these circumstances is to generate gas rather than aid the manipulation of the gluten.

2. The stretching and conditioning of the gluten is achieved through more vigorous manipulation by powerful mixing machines able to achieve the required result quickly.

3. The addition of a small amount of hard fat; that is, fat that will not melt at the temperatures which occur in heavily worked dough. The fat coats and protects the gas bubbles formed and prevents their dispersion before the lattice work is 'set' by heat.

4. The use of emulsifiers to aid the mixing of the ingredients and the dispersion of the fat in the starch gel.

5. Chemical treatments that really have two functions. First, they render the gluten more amenable to mechanical stretching. Secondly, they remove the yellow pigments present in wheat flour thereby making the flour white, traditionally the preferred colour in the UK. (At one time this bleaching was achieved by 'ageing' the flour before use by keeping it for a few weeks during which the oxygen in the air bleached the pigment.) These chemicals usually come in mixtures called 'bread improvers'. Such mixtures include potassium bromate and ascorbic acid (which together form the oxidizing agent that conditions the gluten and removes the pigments), the emulsifiers (permitted by regulation), yeast nutrients and fat (usually lard). We will look at 'bread improvers' again later.

The whole process is highly technical, involving careful control of temperature and humidity during mixing, and temperature and time during cooking. Such control is important if all the reactions are to proceed at just the right pace to produce bread of acceptable quality, weight and freshness.

In some breads, such as soda breads, baking powder is used to generate the gas and no yeast is required. Baking powder is a mixture of sodium bicarbonate and potassium tartrate or some other acid salt. When water is added, the tartrate is converted to tartaric acid, which then reacts with the bicarbonate to produce carbon dioxide (CO_2). These are the ingredients used in self-raising flour, and are commonly employed in cake-making, where the gluten is not manipulated and the final texture more crumbly.

The use of wholemeal flour also affects the gluten treatment so that these breads are less springy and more crumbly than white bread. They can be made more palatable, however, by blending flours with a higher gluten content and by the use of emulsifiers.

The composition of flours and bread is carefully controlled by government regulation. 'Wholemeal bread' must be made only from wholemeal flour and contain not less than 2.2 per cent crude fibre. The now discontinued 'wheatmeal bread' was required to contain not less than 0.6 per cent crude fibre. The term 'wheatmeal' is now illegal and has been replaced by 'brown' so all brown bread must contain the requisite crude fibre. Some brown breads have added caramel to 'improve' the colour and flavour, but there is no truth in the assertion that brown bread is merely coloured white bread. (*See also* p. 135.)

Cakes

Cake batter is an air–fat–water emulsion in which the air phase is stabilized with egg protein and the rest with starch gel. Sugar is dissolved in the water phase and lecithin (from the egg yolk) is used as the emulsifying agent. The 'richness' of a cake is governed by the amount of sugar and fat present, while the aerated state is achieved, first by creating a foam with egg white and then by using a baking powder to generate carbon dioxide during cooking. The skill of cake-making resides in the ability to achieve a stabilized emulsion by means of heated protein at precisely the right moment – that is, when the required degrees of aeration, gas production and gelling occur. The presence of sucrose, and the shorter time involved, prevent the gluten from reacting to the gas production, so that the final texture is not like bread.

In commercial production, the use of emulsifiers is widespread to facilitate large-scale manufacture without the individual control required in the domestic kitchen. Otherwise the process is essentially the same.

Jams

Jams, marmalade and associated jellies are acidic gels of pectin and sucrose with fruit or fruit juice. Originally jam was a means of preserving summer fruit, but nowadays the fruit is preserved and drawn on as required to manufacture jam.

Pectin is another kind of long-chain molecule derived from plants, particularly fruit. Like starch, it forms a gel when mixed with water but with pectin sugar is also necessary. The chemistry of gel formation is very complex but, for simplicity, imagine the chain-like molecules forming a loose network with water trapped in-between. The particular value of pectin lies in its ability to form gels in the presence of the acids derived from fruit and with sucrose molecules as part of the network. The sucrose acts as the preservative because in high concentration (that is above 66 per cent) it prevents micro-organisms gaining access to water.

The commercial manufacture of jam is essentially the same process as that used in the kitchen, except that pectin and citric acid (derived from apples or citrus fruits) are always used because the pectin content of fruit is so variable. The acidity has to be carefully controlled to ensure correct setting. To do this 'buffering agents' such as sodium carbonate may be used. Fruit that has been preserved with sulphur dioxide loses some of its colour. This may be restored with a permitted food colour. In jams specifically for diabetics, with much reduced sucrose, a number of preservatives are allowed. The compositional standard of jams and 'extra jams' with more fruit and less sugar is controlled by government regulation.

Jam is cooked by boiling, sometimes under vacuum, in such standardized conditions that the final product, with reduced water-content, is of a predetermined composition and can be packed into the prepared jars immediately. These are then sealed under partial vacuum, ensuring that the product is sterile. In some jams, ascorbic acid may be used as an antioxidant, and occasionally with curds and marmalades an emulsifier is of value to maintain suspension during cooling and packing.

In reduced-sugar jams, the gel formation cannot rely on sucrose, and chemically modified pectins are used. The resultant gels need to be stabilized with one of the gums or with carboxymethyl-cellulose. In these jams, artificial sweeteners and preservatives are allowed.

Snack foods

To the chagrin of the purists, the snack-food industry continues to advance in range and popularity and perhaps demonstrates food technology at its most developed. Snack foods should not be confused with 'convenience' foods, which are intended as nutritionally wholesome foods presented in a format that is very easily prepared for the table. Thus, fish fingers, canned foods and cooked meats are classic convenience foods. Snacks, on the other hand, are not intended as a main part of a nutritionally balanced diet but are intended to accompany drinks, to quiet hunger pangs between meals, to provide extra energy for growing children or simply as fun.

Most snack foods are composed of wheat starch in the form of semolina (a granular form produced before the final grinding into flour) or of potato starch. The latter is preferred because of its inherently better taste and better frying qualities. Other snack foods include maize (popcorn), nuts, pork rinds, a variety of dips and pastes (toast toppers), a wide range of 'confectionery products' and of course, the ever-popular potato crisp.

Extruders and extrusion cooking play major roles in the manufacture of snack foods. Extruders are machines for forcing a paste through perforated plates, as in the manufacture of pasta. Often this is used as a means of producing a 'half-product' which is then finished (i.e. cooked, coloured or flavoured) by other manufacturers nearer the point of sale.

In extrusion cooking the extruded product is cooked immediately, often by flash-frying. In this case, the mix will contain all the ingredients of the final product, whereas the half-product is little more than extruded starch. The starch base lends itself to the incorporation of flavours and colours to produce wide varieties of snacks. In many cases the final product can be aerated to produce a 'puffed' version: the extruded material is raised to a high temperature so that moisture within it is quickly converted to steam which expands it. Many breakfast cereals are produced by the extrusion cooking process.

Many snack foods have a relatively high content of fat and salt, and are only intended – and packaged – for occasional consumption in small amounts. Snacks are often criticized as if they were intended to be a major component of the diet. No snack, whatever its depiction as a 'healthy' foodstuff, could be regarded as other than incidental to the main diet.

Bottled sauces

A sauce of the type that graces many a British table in bottled form consists of a stabilized suspension of finely divided vegetables and fruits in an acid syrup with added spices. Usually the stabilizer acts as a thickener, increasing the viscosity of the sauce. In thin sauces, no stabilizer/thickener is added so that any solid material sediments and the bottle has to be shaken vigorously (e.g. Worcestershire sauce). The acid is vinegar (acetic acid) and the syrup usually sucrose or glucose syrup, a solution of glucose in water.

In manufacture, the vegetables and fruit are pulped and may need preheating to drive off any sulphur dioxide used as a preservative. All the ingredients, except the stabilizer and spices, are then simmered and stirred until softened. The mixture is then sieved and the stabilizers and spices added. The suspension continues to be stirred and is again sieved. The contents have to be calculated very accurately to ensure that the final viscosity is correct and that the mixture remains suspended but does not gel.

Usually, sauces keep well by virtue of their sugar, salt and acid content, but some preservatives are allowed such as benzoate, sorbic acid or sulphur dioxide – all to defined limits. Added colours such as caramels are sometimes used.

This chapter has dealt with the basics of food preparation, mixing and cooking, and has tried to illustrate how these commonly used processes are adapted to large-scale manufacture. The essential problem, as always, is to obtain a consistent product that the consumer will accept and enjoy. To achieve this a wide range of technical expertise has to be applied. The issue of the inevitable compromise on taste and appearance is dealt with in Chapter 11.

8 Food Preservation

Rotten food is no good to anyone and can be dangerous. What is done and why to keep food wholesome and safe

David M Conning

The techniques of food processing are concerned with preserving food by the reduction of contamination by bacteria and moulds. In this chapter, we look at the food processes designed specifically to preserve food produced on an industrial scale.

Canning

This term primarily refers to foods packed in 'tin' cans but any suitable container would do. Food is sealed in a watertight and airtight container that can then be heated sufficiently to render the contents sterile. In doing this the inherent tendency of foods to degenerate may also be prevented, but not always and the food can spoil. Some canned foods have remained edible for a hundred years – others have not lasted more than a year. Where a canned product is likely to deteriorate within eighteen months, it will be marked with a 'best before' date. In general, it is unwise to keep canned food for longer than a year or so, not because it will be dangerous, but because it may be spoiled. The canning process has several stages.

Preparation The foodstuff is cleaned and all inedible parts are removed. This is done by hand.

Blanching The food, if suitable, is immersed in hot or boiling water, or is steamed. This has a number of effects, the main one being to kill the enzymes that will cause deterioration. Other effects are to drive out trapped air, to shrink the food and to help preserve colour and flavour.

Filling   The food is cooked, chopped, pureed, or suspended in oil or syrup. An important part of filling is the 'exhaustion' of the gap left at the top of the can. It is important that oxygen (which promotes corrosion) should be excluded by steam injection, by the steam from the hot food itself, or by vacuum, especially if the contents are meat or fish. The processes used result in a partial vacuum inside the can after it has been sealed with an end plate that is mechanically seamed into place.

Sterilizing   Where the contents of the can are acidic in nature (some fruit and tomatoes, for example), the filled and sealed cans may be sterilized by immersion in boiling water only. This is because the most dangerous germ, *Clostridium botulinum*, which produces the deadly toxin referred to earlier, cannot survive in acid conditions. Nitrite, present in cooked and cured meats, also kills this bacterium and prevents its spores developing. With other foods, the cans have to be sterilized in a pressure autoclave using high temperature.

Aseptic packing   Where these treatments would result in over-cooking of food, for example with soft fruits, an aseptic technique is used. The cans are pre-sterilized by heat, the food is sterilized (by raising to a high temperature of 149 °C for a few seconds, followed by rapid cooling) and then packed, and the cans are sealed under vacuum. This process has also been adapted for plastic and cardboard containers; pre-sterilization is performed by hydrogen peroxide which is quickly removed prior to filling. Such a process is used, for example, for UHT milk.

Labelling   Finally, the cans are partially cooled, dried (usually by their own heat) and labelled. Commonly, the cans are coded so that they can be readily identified at a later stage if necessary. Some will also be stamped with a 'best before' date.

Cans are usually made from mild steel coated with tin and are often seamless. Seamed cans have double seams with a sealant material embedded in the join. Cans destined to contain acid materials are coated internally with an inert lacquer that is fixed

8.1 Cans and their construction

A three-piece electrically welded food can.

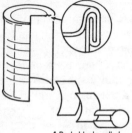

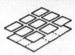

1 Tinplated sheet steel cut on a shear press.

2 Protective coating applied. Printing as customer's specification. Curing.

3 Coated sheets slit into individual body blanks.

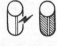

4 Body blanks rolled into cylinders.

5 Overlapping seam welded and a second coat of lacquer.

6 Formed cylinder is flanged at both ends.

7 Cylinder ends punched out of sheet steel.

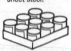

8 End rims curled and a sealing compound applied.

9 One end double-seamed to can.

10 Spray coating on inner surface. Baking and curing.

11 Final testing. Packing.

A two-piece drawn and wall ironed can. (DWI)

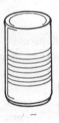

1 Press punches out cups from aluminium or steel.

2 Cups rolled to full length. Bottoms domed.

3 Top trimmed to length.

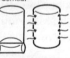

4 Cans thoroughly cleaned.

5 Surface printed to customer's specification.

6 Domed bottom varnished and can baked.

7 Protective inner coating applied. Second baking.

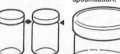

8 Can ends necked to correct size.

9 Ends flanged for future double seaming.

10 Final testing. Packing.

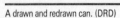
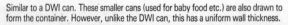

A drawn and redrawn can. (DRD)

Similar to a DWI can. These smaller cans (used for baby food etc.) are also drawn to form the container. However, unlike the DWI can, this has a uniform wall thickness.

by heat during manufacture, which prevents the tin coating from being dissolved. If, as a result of damage to the lacquer, the lining were to dissolve, the concentration of tin that would escape into the food would rarely exceed 40 p.p.m. (parts per million). The current safety limit for tin is 250 p.p.m. so there is a sizeable safety margin. Some lacquers contain zinc. This neutralizes the sulphides that are produced when vegetables and some meats are heated, and cause 'blackening' of the inside of the can. Those destined for highly humid conditions (the tropics) often have the outsides coated with lacquer as well.

In recent years, some non-acid foods packed in unlacquered cans have caused problems because of an increase in the nitrate content in the general water supply. The nitrate oxidizes the tin, causing it to be released into the contents of the can. The increased levels in the food have resulted in one or two episodes of tin poisoning. Tin poisoning causes acute vomiting, and diarrhoea. It is not dangerous but is extremely unpleasant. In the UK the water used for canned foods is controlled for nitrate content, but this may be a continuing problem with products from abroad where water is not maintained to the required standards.

Similar problems may be encountered with some meat products containing nitrite, such as corned beef and ham. These products should always be packed in fully lacquered cans. For some products, such as rhubarb, the acidity is such that even heavily lacquered cans have limited durability (6 to 18 months). Alternatively, steel cans may be used.

Aluminium cans, effectively lacquered, have found widespread use for gassy beverages, mainly because they can be scored for easy opening. They are easily dented, however, making them generally unsuitable for foodstuffs.

Canned foods have become part of our way of life and are rightly regarded as safe and dependable. It is sensible, nevertheless to observe a few simple precautions.

1. Clean the can top before opening. A rinse over with clean water will do.
2. Check whether the can has a date stamp. Do not use out-of-date material and discard all unused cans after a year.
3. Avoid dented cans. The dent may have damaged the internal lacquer.
4. Once the can has been opened, use the contents straightaway. Do not keep unused contents in the can but in a separate

container and make sure they are well re-heated before eating.
Cooked meats kept in a fridge will be alright.

Freezing

At low temperatures, all of the activities that result in food spoilage
– natural deterioration and the activity of microorganisms – are
slowed down considerably. In addition, the water that is present in
the foodstuff, which is an essential part of the chemical reactions
resulting in spoilage, is converted to ice and cannot be used by the
enzymes or the bacteria. If, however, the freezing occurs slowly,
the crystals of ice are large and they themselves damage the
foodstuff, so that on thawing the food may lose a lot of fluid or
become mushy. If freezing takes place rapidly, the crystals are
small and damage is prevented. Thus the processes used in food
freezing are known as quick freezing or accelerated freezing. The
main methods are as follows.

Plate or contact freezing   Used for flat products such as beefburgers,
fish, etc. The food is packed in flat cartons between hollow metal
plates through which a cooling fluid is circulated. The plates are
pressed down on the packed foodstuff during freezing.

Blast freezing   For more bulky products such as meat and baked
goods, the food is passed through a tunnel with a blast of cold air
coming the other way. A more recent version of this is the 'fluidized
bed'. Here the food 'floats' on a cushion of cold air as it passes
down the tunnel. With some products, the cartons are placed on
cold plates and blasted with cold air.

Immersion freezing   The food products are totally immersed in a
cooling fluid after being wrapped in an impermeable film. The fluid
for immersion is normally a solution of calcium chloride or sodium
chloride cooled by refrigeration (the salts prevent the water freezing). With calcium chloride, temperatures down to $-34\,°C$ can be
achieved, with salt, $-18°C$.

Cryogenic freezing   A more recent development has been the use
of liquid nitrogen or liquid carbon dioxide. Because these liquids

only exist at very low temperatures, refrigeration is not needed. To prevent surface-cracking, the products are pre-cooled with liquid nitrogen spray or gas before immersion. Freezing is extremely rapid but the process is expensive to operate. Once frozen, food can be stored for very long periods at temperatures between − 18°C and − 30°C. White fish, for example, will keep for several years at − 30°C. The technique is of particular value for the preservation of vegetables, fruit and fish, but, now that rapid freezing techniques are becoming widely available, it will be increasingly used for a broader range of foodstuffs.

The domestic deep-freeze, of enormous popularity and usefulness, is increasingly used to store prepared meals and cooked products. The freezer's main benefit is its ability to hold foodstuffs in a near 'fresh' state so that the colour and nutritional content are well preserved. It is less suitable for chemically 'raised' foods, such as those made with baking soda, and for cured products containing, for example, nitrate. This is because the chemicals used in these products tend to be concentrated in the freezing process, due to the slight dehydration that occurs. Unpleasant off-tastes can develop as a result.

A star system is used as a guide to storage in the freeze compartments of refrigerators. Deep-freezers will maintain temperatures of below − 18 °C indefinitely and in addition may have a rapid freezing compartment.

Foods kept frozen below − 18 °C will remain safe indefinitely and the duration of storage is governed by the eating quality. This depends on the food, and the purchaser should be guided by instructions at the point of sale. Table 8.2 gives a general guide. A good freezer cookbook will give full details.

Table 8.1 **Star system of storage**

Star rating	Temperature	Duration
*	Less than − 6 °C	7 Days
**	Less than − 12 °C	1 Month
***	Less than − 18 °C	3 Months

Table 8.2 **Storage guide for frozen goods**

Food	Duration of storage (months) at −18 °C or below
Beef	12
Pork	9
Chicken	12
Turkey	9
Duck	6
White Fish	4
Salmon	3
Shrimps	2
Veg (blanched)	12
Bread	1
Cakes	2

Dehydration

The preservation of food by drying has been practised for centuries in countries where there is clear sunshine and little humidity. In unkinder climates, preservation by drying has usually been combined with curing by wood smoke.

Nowadays, foodstuffs may be dehydrated in a stream of hot air or in vacuum driers. Liquids may be 'spray dried', as for example in the production of milk powder (*see* page 85), soups and instant coffees.

Dehydration preserves food by removing the water vital for microorganisms and spores to develop and spoil the food. It does not in itself remove microorganisms or spores. Foodstuffs, therefore, have to be heat-treated in some way prior to drying. Vegetables are either blanched with boiling water or steam, or treated with sulphites; meat and fish are cooked; and liquids are pasteurized (*see* page 82). Where the drying process has involved 'smoking', various chemicals (such as phenols) in the smoke have a disinfectant effect and further treatment is not necessary to render the food safe.

The dehydrated product must be protected from exposure to moisture, high temperatures and oxygen. Moisture obviously results in reconstitution, making the food vulnerable to spoilage. Storage temperatures above about 30°C make dried foods much darker in colour (browning effects), which is not always acceptable to the consumer. Oxygen changes fats and oils, causing rancidity or the development of other off-flavours; it also causes changes in colour, through a bleaching effect, and destroys some vitamins (A and C). Dehydrated foods are also liable to absorb other food odours (cheese, onions) and paint odours.

For all these reasons, dehydrated foods have to be packed in absolutely impervious materials, preferably under vacuum (i.e. with all air excluded from the pack), or in an inert atmosphere such as nitrogen. Modern developments in plastic film and packaging equipment are now able to meet these requirements – at a price. The reconstitution of dehydrated foods is best done if materials other than water can be excluded. Thus gases and other dissolved compounds should be avoided. To achieve this, open the vacuum-packed product while it is immersed in warm water, previously boiled to drive off contaminant materials. Where the material is in powdered or granular form (soups, coffee), these procedures are not required. Such products keep indefinitely and do not require special conditions for storage. Once opened, the product should be used quickly or stored in the fridge for only two or three days.

Freeze-drying

The combination of quick freezing and drying is a technique that holds much promise for the future. If ice crystals are subject to reduced atmospheric pressure and then slightly warmed, they convert instantly to vapour and do not pass back through a liquid phase. It is possible, therefore, to dehydrate frozen food and achieve the advantages of both processes: that is, the food has all the qualitative and nutritional advantages of deep freezing together with the lightness and compact nature of dehydrated foods. At the same time, it can be stored at ordinary room temperatures. The process is expensive, requiring very careful control, but could be a major development for some foodstuffs in future years.

Chemical preservatives

The processes involved in providing food for the consumer are closely under the control of the manufacturer. His control and monitoring techniques are often highly technical. Once in the hands of the retailer or consumer, however, the manufacturer has no further control of the product – how it is stored or handled, or how long before it is consumed.

Were all consumers (and retailers) to possess efficient refrigeration and to observe time (shelf-lives, 'best before' dates) and temperature constraints strictly, few problems would be expected. This is not the case, however, and incorporation of chemical preservatives into certain foodstuffs has become common practice to provide protection, once the product has left the manufacturer.

A good deal of adverse publicity has been given to the presence of chemical preservatives. Bowing to consumer demand, manufacturers and retailers are now marketing products free of such compounds. In these circumstances, it is imperative that the recommended shelf-life and storage conditions are strictly observed. Two types of chemical preservatives are in common use: antioxidants and antimicrobials.

Antioxidants
All fats and oils are susceptible to attack by the oxygen in the air. This results in the formation of breakdown products (called peroxides and aldehydes) which bring about rancidity. All foodstuffs that contain fat or oil are vulnerable to this type of deterioration. Even living creatures, dependent on oxygen and embodying fat, are susceptible to the formation of peroxides and are equipped with enzyme systems to prevent the build-up of such products. These enzyme systems are killed off in food processing to prevent spoilage, so some other means must be found to do that particular job. Several types of chemicals have the ability to absorb oxygen thus preventing its effects on food. These are listed below.

Butylated phenols   There are several in this category including the well-known butylated hydroxyanisole (BHA – E320) and butylated hydroxytoluene (BHT–E321). These compounds are of great value because they can withstand fairly high temperatures without decomposing. They are mainly used in cooking fats and oils but are important in many other products.

8.2 Birth of an E number

The classification of additives by E number is made through a 'Directive' produced by the European Commission. Once classified an additive is then listed in one of two 'annexes'. The first contains additives that must be accepted by all member states. The second contains additives which may or may not be used depending on national circumstances. But all additives with E numbers have to be cleared for safety.

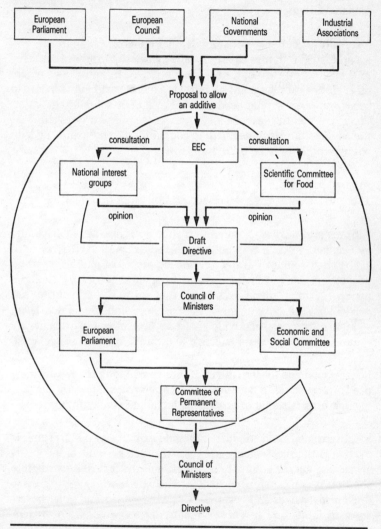

The gallates These are compounds derived from gallic acid, known as propyl, octyl or dodecyl gallates. They are also used in fats and oils, sometimes in combination with BHA and BHT. Butylated phenols and gallates are frequently used with citric acid, which removes the metallic compounds that interfere with anti-oxidant activity.

Naturally occurring compounds Tocopherol (vitamin E) and ascorbic acid (vitamin C) are usually synthesized rather than used in their natural extract forms. They are used in baby foods where other antioxidants are not permitted. Ascorbic acid may be used in beers and other similar products, because of its solubility in water. They are neither as effective nor as temperature-resistant as the phenols and gallates. Other compounds (ethoxyquin and diphenylamine) may be used on fresh fruit.

Antimicrobials

These are chemicals that kill bacteria or fungi (moulds).

Nitrates and nitrites Compounds that were discovered originally by accident when it was noticed that salted meat (preserved with saltpetre or sodium nitrate) developed patches of pink colouration due to the conversion of the salt to sodium nitrite by bacterial action. It was then discovered that nitrate and nitrite are particularly effective against *Clostridium botulinum*. Since then, sodium nitrite has been widely used to protect against this deadly organism, and as yet no effective alternative has been discovered.

Benzoic acid and its derivatives These are among the most widely used preservatives in beverages, jams and syrups. They are effective against a wide range of organisms including some fungi.

Sulphur dioxide and sulphites Despite its pungent odour, sulphur dioxide is the most widely used preservative because of its occurrence as a gas, its solubility in water, and the fact that as sulphite solution it can be sprayed. It is extensively used on fresh grapes, dried fruits, salads and vegetables, in wines, beers and other beverages, in jams, and in cooked meats. Its use dates from ancient times when burning sulphur was a commonly used fumigant. One of its advantages is that residues tend to be removed during cooking, though its widespread use in wine-making may result in persistent, albeit small, concentrations in the final product.

Sorbic acid and propionic acid Valuable because of their anti-fungal activity, these are widely used in cakes, bread, puddings and cheeses. Sorbic acid is tasteless and odourless, whereas propionic acid salts are slightly cheesy (and are used in cheese). Propionic acid is produced by bacterial activity in the digestive tract of cows and occurs naturally in butter. It is of particular value in preventing bread from going mouldy.

Organic acids (citric and acetic) Microbes do not thrive in acid conditions. Thus citric and acetic acids are effective anti-microbials in some circumstances, particularly in canning applications.

Gaseous preservatives To be most effective all the compounds mentioned so far require water to be present. With some crops (e.g. stored cereals) reduced water-content is essential. In these circumstances, gassing by ethylene oxide or propylene oxide is commonly used. They have the added bonus of pest control as well as anti-microbial activity.

The use of all of these compounds is very closely regulated and they may be used only up to certain concentrations, which are very small as a proportion of the weight of food consumed. Furthermore, the limits generally apply to the *total* amounts of anti-oxidants or preservatives present. If more than one is present, the concentrations of individual compounds may have to be reduced.

There can be no question but that the use of preservation techniques, including the use of chemical preservatives, has played a major role in maintaining public health. Neither would such a wide range of food be available to the consumer without them. Chemical preservation has an added advantage over other methods in that they remain with the food until its final preparation (and, to a limited extent, beyond that). They offer some protection, therefore, against unhygienic domestic practices. Nevertheless, it seems likely that, as new industrial techniques are developed, the use of chemicals will decline. When this happens there will be a considerable need for improvement in hygienic standards in kitchens.

Food irradiation

Low-intensity electromagnetic radiations of very short wavelength (gamma rays, X-rays) inhibit the metabolism and interfere with the reproductive division of living biological cells. They pass through tissues virtually unimpeded and are therefore effective at killing bacterial contaminants of foodstuffs. They have been advocated as an effective means of reducing bacterial spoilage, killing those organisms likely to cause disease.

Up to now, the cost of generating the radiation has prevented the widespread use of this technology, but the materials that spontaneously produce radiation of the requisite low intensity (Cobalt–60; Caesium–137) are now both more readily available and cheaper. Therefore, food irradiation is now a feasible addition to the range of preservation techniques. It has been used extensively to sterilize the food of laboratory animals and of those hospital patients in need of protection against any kind of bacterial invasion. In these circumstances, it is known to be perfectly safe. Indeed, laboratory animals tend to thrive better on food sterilized in this way.

As far as can be determined – and extensive research has been carried out – there are no adverse nutritional effects with food irradiation compared with other methods. Changes do occur but these tend to be less, and are certainly no more, than occur with other forms of food processing, such as cooking. Changes in taste occur if the radiation is above a certain intensity but, at the level that would be permitted, such changes appear to be negligible.

Most foods are naturally slightly radioactive because they are grown in (or, in the case of animals, they consume plants that are grown in) soil that contains naturally occurring radioactive materials. At the permitted level of food irradiation, no radioactivity is induced in the treated food. The irradiation process itself would operate well within the known safety levels for workers in the radiation industries. No adverse effects are to be expected from the wider introduction of this technology to food processing.

The advantages are likely to be substantial. Radiation is effective against pathogenic bacteria such as salmonella, the main cause of serious and occasionally fatal food-poisoning, which is particularly common in poultry. Radiation's action against spoilage organisms will undoubtedly help to preserve food for longer periods of time. It is less effective, at the allowable doses, against spores and would be of little use on its own against *Clostridium botulinum*.

The main problem is that it is not possible, at present, to detect that food has been irradiated. It is, therefore, theoretically possible that food that would be condemned on the grounds of micro-biological contamination – but had not deteriorated to an extent that was detectable by appearance, smell or taste – could be rendered apparently wholesome by irradiation. It is conceivable that food treated in this way could contain unacceptable concentrations of bacterial toxins, even though no living bacteria remain.

The main argument, however, rests on the issue as to whether the consumer should be misled into believing that the food is wholesome, merely because the bacterial tests are unable to prove otherwise. It is probably advisable not to permit the use of irradiation for food preservation, until methods are available to ensure that irradiated food is identifiable as such. Within the UK this may be achieved by control and inspection, suitable documentation and labelling. The modern food industry, however, uses food products from all over the world and more safeguards are likely to be needed before such protection can be guaranteed for imported goods.

Food preservation – the future

It seems likely that food preservation in the not too distant future will be enhanced by the addition of irradiation and freeze-drying techniques, provided that they can be suitably controlled, the products adequately packaged and the costs made competitive.

Adequate protection against *Clostridium botulinum* will remain one of the controlling factors on food-preservation techniques, until improvements in food sterilization by heat can be achieved without such drastic, adverse effects on taste. Until then, it is likely that the continued used of nitrite will be required.

Whatever happens in the development of food-preservation techniques, a greater awareness amongst consumers and catering establishments of the dangers of inadequate food and kitchen hygiene is desperately needed. It makes sense to suggest that the principles of good domestic practice should be included in the school curriculum.

9 Additives in Foods

Advanced technology or a cheap fraud? Here are the facts – you can be the judge

David M Conning

Food processing on a large scale involves the use of a wide range of chemical compounds to facilitate and control the various procedures involved, and to safeguard health. Some of these compounds are used in the domestic kitchen where food processing is under the watchful eye of the cook. In industry, where moment-to-moment control is not possible by observation, other methods are used. These increasingly involve computers and the use of automation.

In addition, food science has developed a range of compounds that will carry out a particular function within very narrowly specified limits, thus reducing the possibility of error in some of the delicate processes involved. The manufacturer is thus able to standardize procedures so that his bread, cakes, margarines, sauces and soups will come out the same, time after time.

There can be little doubt that large-scale processing has resulted in some reduction of the aesthetic quality of some foods. Manufactured foods are rarely considered to be as nice as the home-cooked equivalent – though they are getting better. Many feel that this difference also indicates a loss of nutritional quality. This is not true.

All processing, including home cooking, reduces nutritional quality in some ways as we will see in the next chapter, but the gains in nutritional availability from processing far outstrip any losses. It has also to be said that in many instances home cooking leaves a lot to be desired, both aesthetically and nutritionally, so that for some the availability of processed foods represents a real improvement! For those living alone, for the very elderly, and for those with little time to cook, access to processed foods in small portions makes a real contribution to dietary welfare.

The safety of additives worries many consumers. If people believe that their food is 'adulterated' with large amounts of chemicals – *not realizing that all kinds of cooked foods have to use chemicals of some kind* – they believe, at worst, they are being poisoned and, at best, that the manufacturer is cheating them. Emotional reactions, which have been reinforced by many journalists and TV presenters, come to outweigh rational analysis.

Safety

Any chemical used in foodstuffs has to go through a rigorous testing procedure using experimental animals. These tests are designed to detect whether a given chemical mixed in the diet can cause any effect over the lifetime of the animal, and if so, at what dose (i.e. what concentration in the diet) such an effect occurs and what is the highest dose that does not produce the effect. That concentration is defined as the 'no-effect level'.

The usual regulatory practice is to divide that dose by 100 to give a substantial safety margin, and to treat the result as the maximum permitted level of incorporation in the human diet, the so-called acceptable daily intake (ADI). Thus, the maximum amount of any additive that is permitted in the human diet is *at least* 100 times less than the amount known *not* to cause any effect whatsoever when given to experimental animals, usually over a lifetime (i.e. between weaning and death). Often the period of administration is between conception and death, the additive being administered to the parent animal during pregnancy.

In searching for an effect, a wide variety of investigations is undertaken, involving practically the whole spectrum of biological knowledge. As our understanding of biological processes has increased, so the range of tests has expanded. As a consequence, it now costs upwards of £500,000 to accomplish all the tests. The outcome is virtual certainty that, at a specified level of dosing, there will be no adverse effect on any identified biological activity in an experimental animal during its lifetime.

This system is open to criticism on a number of grounds but in respect of human health there are two problems. First, there can be no certainty that the experimental animal is always a good 'model' for human reactions. If the human is very much more sensitive, reducing the permitted exposure 100 times might not be enough. Nor is it established, unequivocally, that a lifetime exposure of a rat, for example, to a chemical (say two years) equates with a lifetime exposure in a human (say seventy years). Furthermore, a human is heir to a number of diseases that do not occur in the rat or other experimental species. Such animals may not, therefore, be good predictors of human susceptibility.

The second problem is that the experimental observations we make are related to our state of biological knowledge: that is, we look for what we know about. Our biological knowledge of the mechanisms of human disease as they occur in the rat is not very advanced. It is possible, therefore, that the investigations undertaken might not be relevant to human disease.

On the face of it these are difficult problems and much has been made of them by people with other axes to grind. It is all too easy to create anxiety in the mind of the consumer by presenting these problems out of context and out of perspective. The fact remains that, for all practical purposes, we can be sure that any biological effect will depend on the size of the chemical dose and, if the concentration of the chemical is reduced sufficiently, no adverse effect will occur. Thus, even the most poisonous of substances can be swallowed with impunity if the dose is small enough. As our regulatory system is designed to ensure that negligible amounts will be eaten, we can be satisfied with it until our understanding of biology has progressed sufficiently to allow more penetrating analyses.

There will be problems. One such is the difficulty of measuring immune effects in animals such as the rat, which appears to be much less advanced than man in respect of this defence mechanism. This may be of particular importance when dealing with allergic reactions to food components and additives. Another problem area is behaviour. It is certainly proving difficult to measure the equivalent of human behaviour patterns in any experimental animal.

But life itself is a risky business and full of much more important uncertainties. If we were to apply our current test procedures to the natural chemicals in food itself, it is likely we would eat very little at all. Certainly, many foods in their natural state would fail such tests. Research is progressing all the time and eventually all the answers will be known.

The compounds added to food can be divided according to their purpose. There are three main groups, plus a small group for specialist applications.

Types of Additives

1. Preservatives, including antioxidants (*see* Chapter 8)
2. Processing aids such as emulsifiers and stabilizers (*see* Chapter 7)
3. Cosmetic compounds that affect colour, taste, sweetness and texture
4. Special effects

Groups 1 and 2 have been dealt with already, so let us take a look at the cosmetic and special agents.

Colours

For those who have access to enough food, colour is very important in helping to decide what to eat. If all food was a uniform grey, like porridge, eating would be tedious. With the possible exception of irradiation, all forms of food processing change the colour of food. Cooked food is not usually as intense in colour as raw produce and sometimes the colours may change dramatically, as in cooked meat, dextrinized starch (which gives the golden colour to cooked pastry), caramelized sugars and the browning reactions. On the other hand, freezing may intensify some colours.

It has been custom for centuries for food-sellers to make their wares more attractive by adding colours. Indeed, food regulations in this country came into being to curtail the use of some colourful but poisonous substances. With the advent of synthetic dyes, about 100 years ago, the regulations became more formal.

Nowadays, to be used in foods, colours, as with all additives, not only have to meet stringent safety requirements but also have to be shown to be *necessary*. Usually, the expert committees that advise the government will not assess the safety data, unless a need for the additive has been established.

The need for a colour is decided on two grounds. One is whether the required effect can be achieved by materials already permitted.

Very often this is possible by using a combination of other, already permitted colours. The drawback, however, with this procedure is that, increasingly fewer and fewer colours are used. Thus the dose of any one colour in the overall diet tends to increase, and that goes against the procedure for regulating safety, which is to keep the dose to the absolute minimum. There is a limit, therefore, to how often this combination route can be followed.

The other ground for deciding need is whether a valuable foodstuff would, or should, be acceptable in its uncoloured form. This is a very difficult decision for a committee to take because of individual tastes in determining food choice. People generally like to have green peas not khaki, red strawberries and cherries not brown, and brightly coloured drinks and sweets. So food processors want to display their wares in the most attractive way and would be keen to use any legitimate means to increase sales. This has sometimes been interpreted as an attempt to sell inferior produce by disguising it. Such behaviour would be illegal as well as immoral and modern practice does not accept it, although it is true that produce of cheaper quality – and price – may be made more attractive with colouring.

The Food Advisory Committee has not addressed this aspect of 'need' other than in broad principle: it has stated it wants to see the use of synthetic colours reduced. If this is generally accepted, we must all learn to accept foods with less attractive colouring. More time and money must also be spent on testing natural colours, for these too are very complex chemicals that can have major toxic properties. In recent years, a good deal of publicity has been given to the allergic reaction of some children to some colours. This point is dealt with in Chapter 5.

Tastes and flavours

That we can smell smells and taste tastes is one of the miracles of nature. Locked up in the nose and mouth is the ability to discern thousands of different flavours, with an accuracy and subtlety that cannot be matched by the most sophisticated analytical equipment. This is even more remarkable when we realize that each separate flavour may be due to the combined effect of several dozen different chemicals in a particular food. Two types of flavouring agents are used in foods. These are the flavouring substances themselves and the compounds that bring out the inherent flavours, the so-called flavour-enhancers.

Flavour chemists, those who try to separate the individual components of a given flavour, must first identify and separate many different compounds. If then they wish to recreate the flavour, they must spend many hours testing different combinations of chemicals at different concentrations until the right blend is found. Obviously this job requires a great deal of expertise and patience.

Flavour is of course extremely important in making food attractive to eat. We all know the difference between tasty and tasteless foods and the difference between good and bad tastes. It is true that taste is subject to individual preference, so that some people relish things others cannot stand, but by and large there is general agreement on what tastes good or bad.

Much of the art of cooking has been directed towards creating attractive tastes through different methods of cooking and the production of, for example, sauces and gravies, which confer special flavours when added to cooked foods. Indeed, the development of the wide variety of tastes that characterize national styles of cooking depends to a considerable extent on the different herbs used to flavour foods. Italian, French, Chinese, Indian and English dishes are easily discernible because in addition to appearance they rely on different methods of cooking and combinations of different herbs and spices to convey typical flavour.

There is, however, an inherent problem. Many of the chemicals that convey flavours are volatile: that is, they tend to disappear in time or if heated, such as when the food is cooked. Also, as time passes, the chemicals interact with each other and with other compounds in the food, so that some tastes disappear and others are created. That is why, for example, cold meat tastes quite different from hot meat, and why re-heated food often tastes different from when it was first cooked.

When food is manufactured on a large scale, it is impossible to bring it to the table in a freshly cooked state. It has to be cooled, packed, stored and, after purchase, re-heated. Thus the flavour may well be very different from the freshly cooked produce and not what the consumer wanted or expected.

For this reason, a large flavour industry has grown up based on the ability to extract flavours and mix them back into processed foods so that the taste resembles more closely the freshly cooked

9.1 Recipe for a flavour

Cherry flavouring. Table of ingredients

Ingredient	Quantity	Status
Maltol	1.00	Nature ident
Vanillin	1.50	Nature ident.
Ethyl Vanillin	0.50	Artificial
Heliotropine	11.50	Nature ident.
Benzaldehyde	1.00	Nature ident.
Toluylaldehyde	2.00	Nature ident.
Acetophenone	0.70	Nature ident.
Flouve Oil	0.60	Natural
Dimethylbenzyl Carbinyl Butyrate	1.00	Artificial
Methyl Heptyne Carbonate	0.70	Artificial
Benzyl Acetate	0.40	Nature ident.
Propylene Glycol	979.10	Solvent
	1000.00	Artificial

This is a typical flavour used on an extensive scale. As can be seen, the bulk of the contents are exactly as occur in nature with the exception of the solvent, itself approved for food use.

product. It has also proved possible to manufacture sauces, and sauce and gravy mixes that can be added to pre-cooked and frozen meals to recapture the original taste.

About 6,000 different compounds have been isolated that are flavours or components of flavour, and they fall into many categories of chemicals. The vast majority of these chemicals are naturally occurring – that is, they have not been invented by man. For example, of the 2,000 or so flavours commonly used in the UK, only four have been invented by chemists and they are not new but mimic natural flavours.

Many of the compounds identified in nature can, however, be synthesized in the laboratory and this is often done in practice because it is cheaper than the laborious process of extraction, and because the flavour chemical is consistent in quality. Its effect can then be standardized and reproduced consistently. These compounds are, of course, identical to their naturally-occurring counterparts but are, all the same, subject to government control. As a result of such enterprise, many different compounds are widely used in food manufacture to achieve the tastes originally inherent in the foodstuffs. In addition, there are some products (e.g. potato crisps) that can be produced with flavours which were inconceivable some years ago. This all adds to the fun of eating.

There has been some concern expressed about the safety of the many flavours in use. Critics have repeatedly said that most of these compounds have not been tested for their biological effects by the conventional methods. There are several reasons why such testing has rarely been undertaken.

The main reason is the potency of the flavours themselves. Extremely small amounts are needed to achieve the required taste effects, so that the commercial production of these very complex compounds is on a very small scale. This means, in the first place, that the amount consumed by an individual is vanishingly small – less than a teaspoonful every year of all the synthesized compounds and the equivalent of a few grains of salt for the four commonly used artificial flavours. Clearly, even the most conservative of expert committees could take a fairly relaxed attitude to dosages as small as this!

In the second place, to test all compounds in use is an impossible task. It would take the entire world's production of any one compound for at least one year to provide enough material to test. The testing itself would involve millions of experimental animals and enormous amounts of time, human effort and money: It is little wonder, therefore, that the testing of these products by conventional tests has a low priority. Each one, however, has been assessed by advisory sub-committees on the basis of their chemical structure, by analogy with other materials and a variety of other criteria, and their reports published.

Flavour enhancers

Although not flavours in themselves, some chemical compounds have the ability to 'bring out' the taste inherent in some foodstuffs and are therefore useful to unmask flavours already present but at low concentrations. There are several substances capable of this effect but only two compounds are commonly used, both of them present naturally in living tissue.

The first is a substance known as *monosodium glutamate* (MSG). This compound, which is a vital constituent of most living cells (indeed, glutamate is present in quite large amounts in human breast milk), has achieved some notoriety because some people believe they react to it in, for example, soy sauce. Such reactions have not been reproducible in carefully controlled trials, but it seems possible that a small number of people are idiosyncratically sensitive to this compound, in much the same way that others react to proteins or colours, or coffee or orange juice. It is not a problem for the vast majority of people. Even those devoted to Chinese food do not consume anywhere near the permitted limit in the UK. This limit is about 7g per person per day. One would have to try very hard indeed to eat more than 2 g in any 24-hour period.

The second substance is *common salt* (sodium chloride). As well as enhancing inherent flavours, salt has the added advantage of acting as a preservative by restricting the availability of water to microorganisms. It is thus a valuable additive for cooked and cooled foodstuffs. One of the concerns over its widespread use is the possibility that excessive consumption causes high blood-pressure. It has been known for some time that people who already have high blood-pressure can benefit from diets low in salt content. The reason remains obscure. What is *not* known is whether salt can *cause* high blood-pressure in people who do not already have the condition. This problem is discussed further in Chapter 5. Increasingly food manufacturers are providing products with reduced salt, which should be of particular value to sufferers from high blood-pressure. Salt-substitutes in which the sodium is replaced by potassium are also available.

The whole question of the impact of taste on dietary preference is now being investigated very intensively. The discovery of what has been described as a fifth basic taste, *umami* (in addition to sweet, sour, bitter and salt) and its interaction with other tastes and with glutamate has revealed that the lack of specific nutrients influences food preference, at least in experimental animals. Much more is now also being learned about the scientific basis for cooking methods accepted for centuries.

Sweeteners and texture

These two are linked together because sugars, and particularly sucrose, not only impart sweetness to foodstuffs, but endow them with a satisfying 'feel' in the mouth. This sensation is hard to define but is a combination of 'body' and 'smoothness'. Most mammals, including humans, enjoy things that are sweet and this tendency seems to be present from birth, though it is still not certain whether it is genetically determined (i.e. inherited) or is induced by contact with sweet things. The fact is that most of us from a very early age learn to enjoy sweetness for its own sake, and many food manufacturers increase the attractiveness of their products by making them sweet.

This creates a problem for some because sugars (i.e. all sugars like sucrose, glucose, fructose, maltose, etc.) contain energy (though less than half the energy in fat) and if more energy is consumed than used in daily activities, the excess is stored as fat. Thus those who take in more energy than they need tend to become overweight, which might lead to the problems dealt with in Chapter 5.

A body of opinion believes that the food industry is doing us a disservice by use of sugar to make food taste the way we like it. Well, you could hardly expect a food manufacturer to want to make his products unattractive, and as most of us are not overweight, it seems logical that the responsibility should lie with the individual consumer. Those who are putting on weight should take more exercise (i.e increase the energy used each day) and reduce energy intake – which may involve cutting back on sweet things, but could also mean eating less fat or starch and drinking less alcohol, depending on the preferred lifestyle.

Sugar is linked with tooth decay. Dental caries is due to particular bacteria that live on surfaces of teeth and are able to produce a protective coating, called 'plaque', that shields them from the cleansing processes in the mouth. They are then able to live in crevices, producing an acid that corrodes the teeth. It seems that these microorganisms make plaque more readily from some sugars than from other carbohydrates, such as starch, and that sucrose is best (or worst!) of all.

What seems to be most important, however, is how often they gain access to the sugar. A frequent 'fix' that keeps up the concentration of sugar in the mouth is better for the bacteria than the occasional 'orgy'. Thus the frequent consumption of sweet snacks, or prolonged and continuous sucking of sweets, without proper oral hygiene, is most likely to encourage dental caries. The latter eating-habit is one that many children most enjoy and unfortunately they are the most susceptible to dental caries. Children should, therefore, be encouraged to eat sweet things only occasionally and

9.2   Dental caries – how it happens

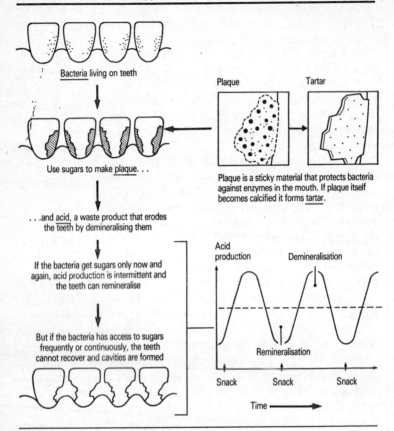

Bacteria living on teeth

Use sugars to make plaque. . .

. . .and acid, a waste product that erodes the teeth by demineralising them

If the bacteria get sugars only now and again, acid production is intermittent and the teeth can remineralise

But if the bacteria has access to sugars frequently or continuously, the teeth cannot recover and cavities are formed

Plaque   Tartar

Plaque is a sticky material that protects bacteria against enzymes in the mouth. If plaque itself becomes calcified it forms tartar.

Acid production   Demineralisation

Remineralisation

Snack   Snack   Snack

Time ⟶

Flouride helps to protect the teeth against the effects of acid.

Three rules for healthy teeth

1. Brush the teeth at least twice a day using a flouride toothpaste.
2. Do not eat sweet or starchy foods or drink sweet or acid drinks more than five times a day.
3. Have a dental check up every six months.

afterwards to clean their teeth properly as well as very regularly.

Since the introduction of toothpastes containing fluoride, the problem of dental caries has declined considerably – though it has not disappeared. Fluoride makes teeth resistant to acid attack but does not reduce the need to remove the bacteria as much and as often as possible; and there is still the need to protect the gums from bacterial attack.

A number of artificial sweeteners have been produced for people who need to reduce their consumption of sugars, but who cannot give up their liking for sweetness. These compounds have the sweet taste (usually they are much sweeter than sugars) but have little, if any, energy content. These are the 'intense' sweeteners (such as saccharin and aspartame) that are used to sweeten drinks or sprinkle on food. They have been of immense value to those who cannot tolerate much sugar at all, such as diabetics, but are also popular with those who are overweight, although their value for such individuals is less certain.

Because of their potential for widespread use, artificial sweeteners have to be thoroughly tested for safety and are carefully controlled by government regulations. As they are very sweet, only small amounts are needed and those that are permitted are known to be very safe and acceptable when used in accordance with the instructions. One, the infamous saccharin, does cause cancer in male rats but only when given in enormous doses to the mother when she is suckling her young – very special circumstances that do not apply to humans.

'Bulk' sweeteners, such as sorbitol or mannitol, are half as sweet as sucrose but can be used to 'fill out' foods from which sucrose has been removed – in other words, to help to restore some of the lost texture.

Special effects

Three sets of additives require separate consideration because of their specialist applications, rather than any particular property they possess. These are the so-called 'bread improvers' and the 'polyphosphates'. And finally, we look at 'hormones' used in meat production.

Bread improvers

For over two hundred years, white bread has enjoyed great popularity compared with wholemeal and brown breads. This arose originally because white bread was associated in the mind of the consumer with a 'cleaner' flour – a flour more likely to be free of dirt and other contaminants (a view for which there was considerable justification at the time).

There was, however, another reason, to do with the texture of the white loaf. When freshly milled, flour has a creamy colour due to the presence of the natural pigments (carotenoids) derived from wheat grain. When the flour was stored for several weeks, this creamy colour disappeared, at the same time changing the flour so that the texture of the baked loaf became more 'springy' and less likely to crumble. This was due to changes in the wheat protein, which are still not fully understood but are probably the result of 'cross-linking' between the molecular filaments of the protein. Such effects were highly prized, and it was common practice for the miller to hold the flour for several weeks before despatching it to the bakers.

It was then found that this 'improvement' in baking quality could be achieved quickly by the use of oxidizing agents, which also decolourized the wheat pigments. Other compounds, such as potassium bromate, were found to bring about the baking improvements but had no effect on the pigments. For some time, flour was treated with a combination of potassium bromate and an oxidizing agent, such as chlorine dioxide or benzoyl peroxide, to bring about the 'ageing' changes quickly. The amounts used were very small (no more than 15 parts per million in flour) and, after baking, the residues were even smaller (all the bromate in fact was converted to bromide, which at these concentrations is innocuous).

More recently, chlorine dioxide has been replaced by another oxidizing agent, consisting of ascorbic acid (vitamin C) and azodicarbonamide. This is supplemented with calcium and ammonium sulphate, to help the yeast to thrive, and with amylase, an enzyme that helps to release maltose from starch.

During the Second World War, all the flour used was obtained by increased 'extraction', that is, to make the flour go further more bran was included. Because bran contains phytic acid, and phytic acid reacts with and binds calcium, it was thought that bread baked with such flour might not provide enough calcium to the

9.3 What's in our bread?

	Wholemeal	Brown	White	Chapati
Protein grams	9	9	8	8
Fat grams	3	2	2	13
Carbohydrate grams	42	45	50	50
Calories (kcal)	216	223	233	336
Fibre grams	8	5	3	4
Vitamin B_1 mg	0.25	0.25	0.2	0.25
Vitamin B_2 mg	0.08	0.06	0.03	0.04
Calcium mg	23	100	100	60
Iron mg	2.0	2.0	2.0	2.0

All figures based on two good slices

diet. By law, therefore, a certain amount of calcium carbonate (chalk) was added to the flour to boost calcium content. After the war, when white bread again became available and the absence of phytic acid removed the possibility of calcium deficiency, the regulation requiring an addition of chalk was maintained to obviate any possibility of dietary inadequacy. White bread is also fortified with iron, and the B vitamins thiamine and nicotinic acid. Wholemeal bread is not fortified in any way.

Polyphosphates

One of the characteristics of meat is that it tends to lose water as the tissues degenerate slightly and the various membranes begin to leak, a process accentuated by freezing and thawing, which is why supermarket meat often sits on absorbent paper. This tendency is inhibited by the salt (sodium chloride) that is present naturally in the tissues. It has been found that the ability of salt to do this is increased by the presence of certain phosphate chemicals, the polyphosphates, and that there are no adverse effects on taste. This is an advantage, particularly with cooked meat such as ham, as the resultant moist texture aids slicing and gives a succulence to the meat.

It has been found, however, that polyphosphates not only protect against water loss but can result in increased water retention, so that more water than necessary could be added to meat without the purchaser necessarily being aware of it. Such a practice would be wholly reprehensible and would indeed render the product 'not of the nature and quality expected', as demanded by our food laws. Although there is no evidence that this abuse occurs in the UK, it seems on balance that regulatory control should be introduced, if only as reassurance. In fact, where water added exceeds 5 per cent, this must be declared on the label, unless polyphosphates have been used, in which case their presence must also be recorded. Several retailers now display the water content voluntarily.

Hormones

It has been the practice for many years to castrate animals intended for meat production. This practice not only results in more docile male animals but causes them to produce more fat. Until relatively recently, meat with a high fat content was favoured because of the much improved taste. At the same time the farmer benefited from the sale of heavier animals. It was known that the same effect could be achieved by the use of female hormones, but as these had to be extracted from glandular tissues they were too expensive for widespread use.

With the development, however, of a synthetic hormone (diethylstiboestrol or DES), increased meat production became feasible and the use of DES became widespread. Usually DES was implanted in some part of the animal that would not be consumed, such as the ear; and in addition, there were other regulations to ensure the absence of any residues by the time the animal was killed. The discovery that DES, in some circumstances, could cause cancer led to a ban on its use in meat production and, regrettably, to illegal black-market sales in Italy, with unfortunate results for some consumers on account of feminizing effects.

The ban stimulated the search for other agents that could increase the carcase weight of animals, and resulted in the discovery of the anabolic agents that are now widely used. These agents act in a complex way, but the effect is similar to growth hormones produced by the pituitary gland, resulting in increased growth of muscle with no excess fat. This increase is very profitable for the farming community and has resulted in a plentiful supply of meat, using fewer animals. It is also an excellent way of producing lean meat.

The use of anabolic agents is strictly controlled and the regulations are designed to ensure that no residues exist in the animals at slaughter. The bad experiences with DES, however, have left a legacy of suspicion on the part of many legislators and some sections of the public, and the EEC has moved to ban the use of all growth stimulators in meat production. The decision is, of course, influenced by the present surpluses, but in the longer term will result in an increased cost of meat. Hopefully, it will not result in the development of another black market where these compounds might also be used in an uncontrolled fashion.

The control of additives

If we are to continue to enjoy the wide variety and convenience of processed foods, and if we recognize that nearly all foods require some form of processing to make them edible, we have to accept that some food additives are essential. It is very important, however, that the additives used are actually necessary and safe. We could not accept a situation where we were in danger of our foodstuffs being adulterated by large numbers of added chemicals, merely for the convenience of the producer, or where we were vulnerable to an unscrupulous manufacturer.

For this reason there has developed, over many decades, a world-wide network of government regulations, established on the advice and recommendations of expert committees, that effectively controls the use of additives. As new information becomes available, so these regulations are reviewed and the use of additives modified; sometimes to allow more, usually to allow less. As food technology advances and newer processes are introduced, there is a tendency to reduce our dependence on chemicals. But this has to be done cautiously to avoid the reappearance of health problems that were once common but are now often forgotten.

At the same time, it is important that people should be aware of what goes into their food, not because they need to be worried about it, but because each of us has to realize how much we depend on our chemical expertise, in order to learn to live with it and to be responsible for deciding how much we allow it to impinge on our own lives. For these reasons, governments throughout the world have sought to inform consumers by ensuring that adequate data are given with the foods they buy, either on labels or in leaflet form.

In Europe, the system of E numbers has been introduced to indicate the presence of additives that have been thoroughly tested and accepted by expert committees throughout the EEC. This system, which is an attempt to avoid the use of cumbersome chemical names, has been misrepresented by some as an attempt to hide from consumers what they have a right to know. Nothing could be further from the truth. It is up to all of us to learn how to use the system to look after our own affairs. There are now many publications, both governmental and private, that explain the position in detail; there are many sources of advice and explanation. No one need be fearful, provided that they are prepared to ask the questions. A list of E numbers appears at the end of this book.

This is not to say, however, that chemical additives should be tolerated without question. Where they no longer serve a useful purpose, they should be removed. We should be constantly vigilant

Table 9.1 **How additives are cleared for use in the UK**

1. Proposal presented to MAFF
May arise as
    (i) part of general review
    (ii) new group of additives
    (iii) modification of current regulation requested

$$\downarrow$$

2. Submitted to Food Advisory Committee (FAC) which
determines whether the additive is needed because
    (i) other additives not suitable
    (ii) there is a consumer benefit
    (iii) a new product needs a new additive
    (iv) there is an economic advantage
If yes,

$$\downarrow$$

3. Committee on Toxicity of Chemicals in Food, Consumer
Products and the Environment (COT) considers

Advice from experts on genetic toxicity and carcinogenesis where appropriate

Data provided by industry, independent research associations published works, WHO/FHO Joint Expert Committee on Food Additives, EEC Scientific Committee for Foods, and other international regulatory organization

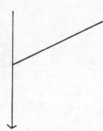

4. FAC Report published with recommendations and comments
invited.

$$\downarrow$$

5. Regulations proposed. Further consultations.

$$\downarrow$$

6. Law into being

Table 9.1 (cont.)

7. The proposal can be rejected at any stage whereupon no
further action is taken.

The COT classifies compounds into one of five categories:

   (i) Acceptable

   (ii) Provisionally acceptable pending more data to be supplied
in certain time period

   (iii) Not acceptable until more data available

   (iv) Not acceptable as data suggests toxicity

   (v) Available data inadequate to decide

9.4 How much artificial flavouring do we consume?

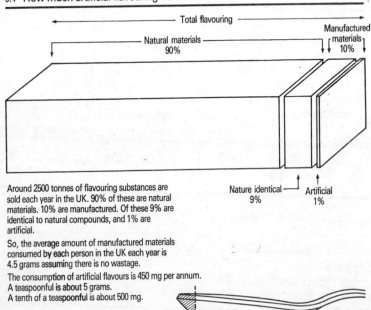

Around 2500 tonnes of flavouring substances are
sold each year in the UK. 90% of these are natural
materials. 10% are manufactured. Of these 9% are
identical to natural compounds, and 1% are
artificial.

So, the average amount of manufactured materials
consumed by each person in the UK each year is
4.5 grams assuming there is no wastage.

The consumption of artificial flavours is 450 mg per annum.
A teaspoonful is about 5 grams.
A tenth of a teaspoonful is about 500 mg.

to ensure that safe limits are not exceeded. In calculating this, the whole diet must be taken into account. However, as individual diets vary so much it is very difficult, if not impossible, to work out how much any one person consumes.

An easier approach, though still difficult, is to measure the total amount being used by the food industry and then to work out what goes into the average diet. Such calculations suggest that, on average, people who live on nothing but processed foods and drinks consume about one-fifth of a level teaspoonful of additives every day of their lives. As about half of the additives used are naturally-occurring compounds, the amount of synthetic additives is extremely small and, given the safety regulations, will cause no problems. Nevertheless, even these small amounts are too much if the additives are unnecessary.

10 Nutritional Effects of Processing

Much ado about very little

David M Conning

Any kind of food processing is intended to increase the palatability of raw foodstuffs, whether by increasing their edibility, or by the prevention of spoilage. It may be stated as plain fact that *any* treatment of food that involves heating will reduce the content of some nutrients. Similarly, any form of prolonged storage results in reduced nutrient content, though the reduction is much reduced at low temperatures.

It is important to understand what is meant by this. Nutrients such as carbohydrates, proteins and fats are certainly changed by cooking or industrial processing but the change usually involves breaking them down into their component parts. The changes are very similar to those that occur during digestion. (*See* Chapter 4 for more detail.) It would be going too far to describe cooking as a form of pre-digestion, but the changes are in that direction. This is one of the reasons why cooked food is more edible. Thus the nature of these types of nutrients is changed, but their nutritional value is not – indeed it may be slightly improved.

Other nutrients are minerals and vitamins. Minerals, by their nature, are not affected by the processing of raw foodstuffs. In fact, the mineral content may be increased by materials derived from the cooking utensils. It is quite common for the levels of iron and aluminium in food to be increased if it is cooked in an iron or aluminium saucepan. It would not be possible to get an overdose as the levels are so low. It *is* possible that some minerals are removed with water but the effect is negligible.

The most important nutrients that are lost during cooking and processing are the vitamins, which are either soluble in fat and oils, or in water. When foods are heated, they tend to lose fat and water.

The vitamins themselves are not necessarily destroyed, but leach out with meat juices or into the vegetable cooking water. If, subsequently, the juices or vegetable water are used for making gravy, sauces or soups, much of the lost vitamin is again available to the consumer. It is thus a good principle in cooking to adopt this practice. Not only are the vitamins recovered, but many of the soluble flavours can also be re-captured. An exception to this rule is in the cooking of various dried beans. These are boiled to destroy toxic or undesirable substances that are naturally present and the water used is best discarded. For example, raw soy beans contain trypsin inhibitors which limit the ability of this enzyme to digest proteins. Broad beans contain vicine, which in some people can cause a condition known as favism. This shows up as a type of anaemia.

Some vitamins are particularly susceptible to destruction by cooking processes. The normal function of these vitamins (C and B_1) is to react with oxidizing compounds that would be damaging if released within living cells, or take part in energy changes in the body. During the cooking process, the vitamins readily react with the available heat and oxygen, and the amount present is reduced. Food processes such as curing and freezing result in similar losses, largely due to the heat treatments used in cooking or 'blanching'.

There is continued loss of vitamin C during storage, though this is less with canned or deep-frozen products than with products kept at room temperature or only slightly chilled. The amount of vitamin lost varies with the foodstuff and with time. For example, tinned spinach may lose as much as two-thirds of its original vitamin C (though on average it is about one-half) whereas tinned asparagus rarely loses more than one-fifth. Green beans lose about a half, whereas peas lose less than a third.

The losses through freezing, where the only heat treatment is blanching, tend to be less, though further losses occur when the food is subsequently cooked. In general, freeze-drying (*see* Chapter 8) is the most effective process as regards vitamin retention, with losses rarely exceeding 10 per cent before cooking. Freeze-drying, which, as its name suggests, involves pre-freezing the food and then drying it, has been widely used in the preparation of soups and instant coffee. Although it is potentially a good way of retaining vitamins, its applications are limited.

Do losses of nutrients through food processing matter? To answer that question we have to do two things. The first is to recognize that what matters is the absolute amount of the vitamin we should be consuming each day. It really does not matter how much of a vitamin is lost from the foods we cook, as long as there is enough remaining in the diet to cover our needs. That depends very much on the individual – and the variation between individuals is tremendous. Governments have issued lists of recommended daily allowances (RDA) which are likely to meet the needs of most people for some nutrients. An example from the World Health Organization is given in Table 10.1. (*See also* Chapter 12, Table 12.1.) This can only be a rough guide because many individuals actually need a lot less. The second thing we have to do is to work out how much of the food in its natural raw state we would consume, compared with the amounts we eat in the cooked or processed forms (Table 10.2)

For most vegetables, there is no comparison. We undoubtedly more than make up for the loss of vitamins by the increased range and weight of foods consumed. For fruits the reverse is the case. If we ate nothing but cooked fruits, we could expect to experience a nett loss of vitamin C intake. For meat, fish and poultry the question does not arise for most of us, as these foods are rarely eaten in their natural state. It is worth noting that where, for example, butter or margarine is used as a cooking medium for meats, there is a substantial gain in the availability of vitamins A and D.

There have been some reports of vitamin D deficiency among some Asian groups living in the UK. The main source of vitamin D is the action of sunlight on the skin and the reported deficiencies have resulted from the use of traditional clothing that shields the

Table 10.1 **Recommended daily allowance (RDAs) of vitamins**

	Vitamins					Calcium	Iron
	A (mg)	D (mg)	B₁ (mg)	B₂ (mg)	C (mg)	(mg)	(mg)
Adult Male	750	2.5	1.2	1.8	30	500	9
Adult Female	750	2.5	0.9	1.3	30	500	28
Children 7–9	400	2.5	0.9	1.3	20	500	10

Source: World Health Organization, Monogram Series, No. 61

Table 10.2 Nutrient loss – vitamins A, D, B, and C per 100 g food

	Raw A (g)	D (g)	B₁ (mg)	C (mg)	Cooked A (g)	D (g)	B₁ (mg)	C (mg)
Flour – wholemeal	0	0	0.46	0	0	0	0.26	0
white	0	0	0.31	0	0	0	0.18	0
Rice	0	0	0.08	0	0	0	0.01	0
Spaghetti	0	0	0.14	0	0	0	0.01	0
Milk – whole fresh	35	0.03	0.04	2.0				
skimmed fresh	Tr	Tr	0.04	2.0				
whole sterilised					31	0.02	0.03	0.8
Egg – whole	140	1.75	0.09	0	140	1.75	0.08	0
Beef Brisket	Tr	Tr	0.05	0	Tr	Tr	0.04	0
Chicken	Tr	Tr	0.1	0	Tr	Tr	0.06	0
Fish – white (cod)	Tr	Tr	0.08	Tr	Tr	Tr	0.08	Tr
fatty (herring)	45	22.5	Tr	Tr	49	25	Tr	Tr
Beans Butter	0	0	0.45	0	0	0	0	0
Cabbage Savoy	0	0	0.06	60	0	0	0.03	15
Carrots	0	0	0.06	6	0	0	0.05	4
Lentils	0	0	0.5	Tr	0	0	0.1	Tr
Peas	0	0	0.32	25	0	0	0.25	15
Potatoes	0	0	0.11	20	0	0	0.08	10
Apples	0	0	0.04	15	0	0	0.03	12
Blackberries		0	0.03	20	0	0	0.03	15
Liver	14,600	0.25	0.21	18	17,400	0.25	0.27	13

Sources: M. Rechcigl Jnr (Ed.) *The Handbook of Nutritive Value of Processed Food*, CRC Press Inc., 1982; R. S. Harmis and E. Karmas (Eds.) *Nutritional Evaluation of Food Processing*, AVI Publishing Co., Inc., 1975; Campden Food Preservation Research Association, 1987.

Note: The concentrations of vitamins in foods is very variable depending on source, season, age and cooking method. The values in this table are illustrative of average results. Tr = trace skin from exposure to the sun. Those wishing to retain this mode of dress should ensure an adequate consumption of eggs and fatty fish.

Although we can conclude that any form of food processing reduces the amount of some vitamins, on balance this has little or no effect on the nutritional content in respect of any other component. The loss of vitamins is counteracted by the increased amounts we are able to eat of processed rather than raw foods. The only notable exception to this rule is fruit and, as most fruit is a good source of vitamin C, fresh fruit should be included in our diet as often as possible. As always, to ensure getting all the nutrients needed, eat as wide a variety of foods as possible. If we do this, expensive supplements will not be necessary.

One final point. It is possible that some old people through neglect, or physical disability, do not eat as much as they should and run the risk of certain nutrient deficiencies. All of us have a responsibility to ensure that our elderly relatives and acquaintances are properly looked after, and do not run the risk of undernourishment.

11 The Aesthetics of Processed Food

The good, the bad and the ugly; and what needs to be done about it

Lis Leigh

Over the past few years, there have been significant changes in what we eat, how we eat and when we eat. Technology has given us food processors, computerized ovens, microwaves and safe chilled or frozen storage for every perishable product. An enormous range of foods has been developed, often geared specifically to technology rather than to taste. We tend not to follow set meal-times, snatching food on solitary occasions. The all-year availability of foods has blurred the impact of the changing seasons. Many of the traditional skills, involving discernment and understanding about foods in their raw and cooked state at different times of the year, have been neglected in the name of convenience.

The emphasis on convenience has left the door wide open for manufacturers to produce whatever will sell; there is probably a greater gap now between the appalling and the good than there ever has been. More foods are now actually manufactured than at any time since processing began. From 1985 to 1986 alone, nearly 400 new 'ready meals' were launched on the market, from Roast Beef Platter (the complete Sunday dinner), to moussaka, cannelloni and chilli con carne. Many of us, however, feel vaguely guilty that the kitchen is no longer a spacious, homely place characterized by inherited skills, the aromas of cooking and the individual creations of the cook, but has been reduced to a small row of cupboards and essential equipment for storing or re-heating.

The reaction to this situation has taken several forms. Attitudes towards manufactured food range from indifference, concern about its effect on health, to an obsession with 'real, natural, country' products, where anything processed is banished from the kitchen.

Food manufacturers are now prepared to respond to health demands, some seeing a policy of reducing additives, adding fibre, and lowering fat and sugar as a supplementary sales tactic, others as a way of maintaining sales. If, as surveys tend to show, half the population believes that 'healthier' eating is the goal to be achieved, manufacturers are prepared to change their products, and introduce new ones, to satisfy this demand.

Technology is developing rapidly, with the increasing use of chill cabinets to control temperature, gas packaging and efficient refrigerated distribution to maintain freshness, and this means that the use of some preservatives can be reduced. Using natural flavours and relying on 'natural' additives adds very little to the cost of the end product.

Whatever the pros and cons of the health debate, it has tended to obscure how we perceive the *quality* of manufactured food. Inferior products can now be sold merely on a supposed health advantage. Health-food shops, formerly somewhat dubious places with sullen assistants, inadequate hygiene, and dusty advertisements claiming miracles for over-priced vitamins and minerals, are now booming and have acquired a self-promoted respectability. Some health-food shops have gone one step further. Realizing that 'healthy' food has become associated in our minds with 'real' food, they have started stocking products formerly found at the grocer or baker.

The emphasis on 'real' and 'healthy' food is in danger of obscuring what is happening in the supermarkets. There are some which sell fresh fish, whole farmhouse cheeses and freshly baked bread, but look at the huge area of a major supermarket, and you will find shelves packed with products that are decidedly inferior aesthetically. Anyone who doubts this should buy a plastic wrapped white sliced loaf, dehydrated soup, some frozen chicken to go with a packet sauce, canned beef, an instant pudding mix and serve it all up for dinner. For many, it will not leave a pleasurable sense of well-being.

Although manufactured products are periodically tested and assessed by an assorted team of 'experts' in newspaper and magazine articles and in television programmes, the criteria used are different from the judgements given by a master chef for restaurant food. It may be possible to rate one product above the others, but to employ the highest standards would entail rejecting them all. It seems to be accepted that there is one rule for the manufacturer and the food technologist, another for the home cook or restaurateur. On the rare occasions when challenged by those who have spent their whole lives practising and experimenting with the taste, flavour and presentation of food, manufacturers will insist that such judgements are specialist, indicative of a 'foodie' minority, middle-class or irrelevant to 'what we know people really like'. If it sells, it must be good – or at least good enough – runs the argument.

Consumer indifference has played its part in the neglect of standards, but it has not been helped by the traditional reticence of the food industry. Secrecy has been justified on the grounds of commercial competition. If X brand is a top seller, then Y will come along, copy it, and dominate the market by selling it for a penny less. Other sectors of industry have learned to live with market competition, whereas the food industry, not least because of the relatively low profit margin it receives, has preferred to keep silent, sheltering behind advertising agencies and public relations companies. The result has been to fuel public distrust and to allow misinformation to run riot.

The story of soup

How, then, does a food manufacturer decide what to make and what to put in his recipe? What exactly are the compromises which have to be made? From which standpoint can we legitimately make a judgement on what he has produced?

Let us take a relatively straightforward food. The instantly heatable can of soup was the first widely popular convenience food, and when the late American artist Andy Warhol reproduced a Campbell's soup can, it was a more potent image to urban society than bowls of fruit or hanging pheasants. Campbell's soup cans are still to be found in every small grocer's and supermarket, even though convenience food, through advanced technology, has become far more ambitious.

The senior soup in Britain is not made by Campbell's, but by Heinz. In 1910 Heinz first introduced their 'Cream of Tomato Soup' from America, and it was manufactured in Britain twenty years later. This must be the most popular soup ever produced, even though it bears little relation to a soup made with fresh tomatoes at home. When it first appeared, canned soup was a luxury product, selling for the equivalent of a servant's weekly wage. Its prestige was based on something we have grown used to: this soup could be eaten safely at any time of the year.

Baxter's of Speyside, manufacturers of canned soups, started life as a small family firm. The managing director, Gordon Baxter, was very partial to his wife Ena's cooking. She made her soup from old family recipes, which exemplified domestic cooking as opposed to the grander style of French cuisine, introduced by Mary, Queen of Scots. Ena Baxter's recipe for vegetable soup was as follows:

Ingredients

2 oz wheatflour	1 bay leaf
8 oz diced carrots	1 sprig thyme, or half tsp. mixed
9 oz diced potatoes	herbs
9 oz diced turnips	half tsp. pepper
7 oz chopped onions	half tsp. salt
1 oz chopped leeks	4 pints strong vegetable or chicken
5 oz sliced carrots	stock; or bouillon cubes
3 oz sliced celery	2 oz butter
2 oz peas	

Method

Sweat the vegetables slowly in melted butter until golden. Add stock and spices. Bring to the boil and simmer gently until vegetables are soft. Mix the flour with a little of the hot stock and add to the soup. Bring back to the boil to thicken. Serve with plenty of crusty wheatmeal bread. Chopped chives may be sprinkled on top and grated cheese added for additional garnish.

The first task was to try to transfer Ena's recipe to a can. The result was disastrous, thick and mushy, the flavour unacceptable. The vegetable ingredients were unrecognizable. The idea seems logical – to capture what is enjoyed at home inside the confines of a can – but in practice, finding the right formula, even with the same ingredients, took a long time.

The major problem lies with the canning process itself. In order to preserve anything in a tin, strict sterilization procedures have to be observed, and this means subjecting the contents to temperatures sufficiently high to kill all bacteria, particularly those capable of causing food poisoning. The most serious form is botulism. These bacteria can only be killed by the high temperature associated with pressure cooking. No simple domestic cooking process can eliminate them. (*See also* Chapter 7.)

The process of sterilization effects profound changes in foods. Colour is lost, texture is altered, and flavours are modified so that they either disappear or become unpleasant. The biggest challenge for a manufacturer of tinned foods is to try to capture the freshness and individuality of a foodstuff.

The transition from home cooking to can involved making radical decisions. First, there was the wheat flour in the original recipe which gives a little body to the soup without unduly thickening it. At sterilizing temperature, wheat flour breaks down, an effect that continues in storage to give a thin, watery soup. The use of a small proportion of corn starch stabilizes the wheat flour and makes the soup shelf-stable without too much thickening taking place.

A second radical change also had to be made. When making vegetable soup, every traditional recipe will specify sweating the diced vegetables first in butter (or some kind of fat) to give richness and flavour. In the canning process, heating in butter results in discoloured, over-soft vegetables in the finished soup. So, instead of adding all the softened vegetables sweated in butter, the butter was used only to cook the onions and leeks, which were added to the stock with the herbs. The carrots, potatoes, turnips and peas would go into the stock raw.

The chicken base of the stock base had to be discarded when vegetarian consumers wrote in complaining that they loved vegetable soup but would not eat animal products. The vegetarian market was becoming lucrative and could not be ignored. Although a fish- or meat-stock base is fundamental to a classic vegetable soup, giving added body to the flavour, it had to go. The garnish, which is always a last-minute addition (if cooked with the soup contents, it would lose its flavour), was also banished. Now that these major characteristics of a good vegetable soup had fallen by the wayside, what was left?

Three ingredients remained which might retrieve the soup from mediocrity: first, prime-quality vegetables, second, a good vegetable stock, and third a successful blend of herbs and spices which might lend distinction. With the help of food technologists and micro-biologists working together in their experimental kitchen, Gordon and Ena Baxter eventually came up with the formula that they

11.1 How Baxters vegetable soup is made

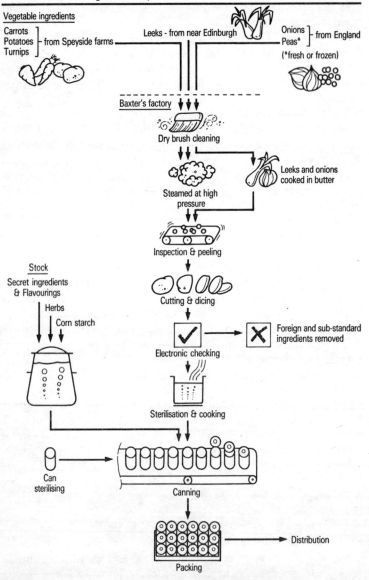

Vegetable ingredients

Carrots
Potatoes – from Speyside farms
Turnips

Leeks - from near Edinburgh

Onions
Peas* – from England

(*fresh or frozen)

Baxter's factory

Dry brush cleaning

Steamed at high pressure

Leeks and onions cooked in butter

Inspection & peeling

Stock

Secret ingredients & Flavourings

Herbs

Corn starch

Cutting & dicing

Electronic checking

Foreign and sub-standard ingredients removed

Sterilisation & cooking

Can sterilising

Canning

Packing

Distribution

thought would be pleasing and successful. And so it proved, in terms of sales. As a consequence, the relative proportion of vegetables, the ingredients of the stock and the exact flavourings are known only to the Baxters and their employees. To reveal this, they feel, would play into the hands of their rivals who have already tried to copy them.

The manufacturing of soup in bulk is a mammoth leap from the contents of a domestic saucepan. The process starts with the arrival of the vegetables. Carrots, potatoes and turnips are grown on farms near the Baxter factory in Speyside, leeks are brought in from other parts of Scotland, celery from near Edinburgh, onions from England. English peas are obtained fresh when in season, frozen if not, as is the case with leeks. Once unpacked from their boxes, the vegetables are put through a cleaning process of dry brushing to remove dirt, stones and other foreign material. They are then steamed at high pressure for a short time so that the skins can be removed, and immediately plunged into cold water to cool. At this point, root-vegetables join other vegetables in passing on to long inspection belts where they are scrutinized for blemishes, and hand-trimmed or peeled as required.

The next stage is to slice, dice or cut the vegetables into different shapes, to create a variation in appearance. Finally the hand-care of the production staff is supplemented by automatic electronic-eye sorting machines, together with magnets and metal detectors and gravity separaters to ensure freedom from foreign material.

The vegetable stock, flavoured with herb essence and added flavours, is made separately in vast cooking kettles holding sufficient liquor for 3000 cans of soup. Fresh and dried herbs have a high bacteriological count and so must be very carefully selected and laboratory-checked before use. The prepared vegetables are then filled fresh and raw in measured quantities into the cans, and the appropriate quantity of seasoned stock added immediately prior to sealing and sterilizing the can.

Whilst all the contents are being heat-sterilized, taking about ten minutes, they are stirred mechanically to ensure they are all cooked at the same time. The relatively short heating period aims at preserving maximum colour and freshness, for in this recipe no flavour enhancers, such as monosodium glutamate (popular because it enhances the natural flavour of canned foods) or colour-additives are used. At this point the mixture is ready for canning.

Once in a tin, labelled and distributed to shops, the contents of the vegetable soup remain stable for a year without deterioration. When opened by someone in search of a quick, hot snack, the contents will be tipped into a saucepan and heated up. The re-heating will destroy some of the original flavour, but as con-venience, rather than taste, is the major factor in choosing tinned soup, flavour will be secondary.

The fact that Baxter's have used prime vegetables, spent years perfecting their recipe, employ an army of quality-controllers and tasters, has resulted in a golden liquid with the vegetables individ-ually distinguishable by texture and shape, if not by flavour. The product is safe, not unpleasant, and able to reduce hunger pangs. The sad fact is, that is probably what most people expect of manufactured food. This product is a good example of its kind, and has more natural flavours than its rivals, but as a vegetable soup, it leaves a lot to be desired.

All cooking, however, is the art of the possible, dependent on which ingredients are available, how many are involved in pre-paration, which kitchen equipment is to hand and what limits there are to the budget. Even within these boundaries, it is possible to look at manufactured food and ask questions which any chef drawing from a pool of inherited skills might ask.

Why, for example, does Campbell's Golden Vegetable Soup contain carrots, potatoes, tomatoes, starch, celery, green beans, peas, sweetcorn, salt, rice, wheatflour, vegetable oil, dried spinach, sugar, hydrolysed vegetable protein, spices, yeast extract, flavour-ings and the colour carotene?

Heinz, with their vegetable soup, have added pearl barley, tubetti (small pasta) instead of rice to bulk out the vegetables, in this case carrots, onions, potatoes, peas, tomato puree and haricot beans. To make this incongruous mix blend together, Heinz have used modified starch, sugar, salt, flour, vegetable oil, hydrolysed veg-etable protein, sodium glutamate (flavour–enhancer) spices and herbs.

Crosse and Blackwell, not to be outdone, sell two vegetable soups: Garden Vegetable Soup and Harvest Thick Vegetable Soup. The first one is bulked out with sweetcorn, beans, and relies on flavour-enhancers and yeast extract. Apart from the standard, and cheap, ingredients, namely carrots, potatoes and onion, the second one goes to town with a fantasia of lentils, pearl barley, wheatflour, beans, dried peas, sweetcorn, yellow pea flour, not to mention flavour-enhancers and the colouring beta carotene. Any half-way decent chef would run out of the kitchen confronted with such an ingredients list!

The real thing

It could be argued, though no manufacturer would be so bold, that if we expect to open a can and experience the taste of a classic vegetable soup, we are fooling ourselves. The constraints of manufacture have led to technology-based 'creations'. As though accustomed to the print of a famous oil-painting never seen, we get a distant reminder of the real thing and forget the identity of the original.

Canned peas are nothing like fresh peas picked from the pod, but canned peas have become so popular that they have acquired an identity of their own. Similarly, 'constructed products' like baked beans or tinned spaghetti have entered the gastronomic experience of most of the population. The problem is not that they are in themselves bad (after all, much home cooking is bad), but that they may be taken for the real thing. As a major part of our school and university life is spent in determining the false from the true (it is still considered a crucial human activity), why not subject the perception of food to the same scrutiny?

On the whole, the majority of manufacturers ignore culinary tradition in the cause of cheapness and novelty. There are many examples. One is the pizza. No matter that the pizza is a proud national Italian dish. Change the dough, a bread base is easier, leave out the fresh tomato sauce, stick on some manufactured tomato paste, make a thin topping of cheap un-Italian cheese like Edam, mixed with a substitute cheese, omit the anchovies because some people do not like them, and sprinkle with dried parsley. The traditional basil is too expensive and who will notice the difference anyway?

If it sells well, develop the line. With a minimal change of ingredients, make a choice of different pizzas, to expand the market. Sausage pizza, with tiny sausage pieces on top, tuna pizza (one of the few fish the British will eat), a vegetarian pizza or a 'healthy wholemeal' pizza. In the fullness of time, the pizza market will be saturated, for everyone will be doing it.

Try something else. Mexican tortillas? Chinese Dim Sum? If

11.2 Profile of a pizza

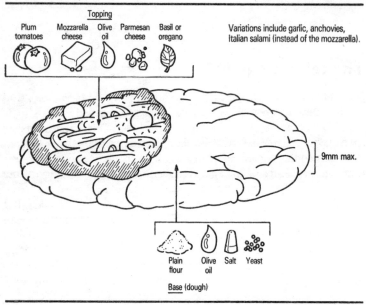

Topping

Plum tomatoes · Mozzarella cheese · Olive oil · Parmesan cheese · Basil or oregano

Variations include garlic, anchovies, Italian salami (instead of the mozzarella).

9mm max.

Plain flour · Olive oil · Salt · Yeast

Base (dough)

existing technology cannot cope with a new ethnic find (all the buyers are travelling nowadays) take the idea and make it British. Anglo-Chinese pancakes. Anglo-Mexican hamburgers. Spices and unfamiliar flavouring can cover a multitude of sins, and if they do not prove popular, a little Worcester sauce will always work wonders . . .

Another example is fruit squash. There are compositional regulations governing the amount of fruit that has to be included in squashes, fruit drinks and juices, and what a manufacturer may call his product – but within this there is wide flexibility. With the appearance of competing products in the market, and the demands of supermarkets who prefer basics like this to be cheap (particularly the case with 'frontline' products consumed in quantity by children), a manufacturer could only keep an edge on competitors by lowering the price. The easiest and cheapest way to do this is to cut back on expensive ingredients, rather than to invest in more automated equipment to increase efficiency, or spending less on advertising which could be seen as self-defeating. The three steps to a squashless squash are as follows:

1. Cut down the amount of fruit.
2. Remedy the reduction of natural fruit flavour by adding concentrated, artificial flavour.
3. Add more sugar.

Since hardly anybody nowadays squeezes fruit to make squashes, there is no constant reminder of what a fresh fruit juice should really taste like. A sweet, rather than fruity, taste is what we, and particularly children, have come to expect in bottled drinks.

The substitution of fruit by flavouring and an increased sugar content is not an overnight process. The first time the fruit content is reduced slightly and the sugar increased a little, even a professional taste-panel will notice no change. If you repeat the process once or twice a year for, say, five years, the changes in the recipe will be graded imperceptibly so that in the end the memory of the original product will be forgotten. If, by chance, a drink made with fresh lemons or oranges is tasted on a trip abroad (many European bars still use a fruit-squeezer) it is possible that it could actually be a shock to the taste-buds, too sour and full of unwelcome bits of fruit.

The difficulty here is that the conditioning effect of constantly having the manufactured version – cheap, convenient and always available – has turned into a preference. If the original does not exist for fairly constant comparison, and has not existed for a period of time, the manufactured copy will no longer seem artificial. The 'fruit drink' has for some become 'sweet coloured stuff out of a bottle'.

Other foods have also undergone a cheapening metamorphosis. There are many regulations covering compositional standards of foods (though some new products are not covered by the existing rules), and some manufacturers use the lowest allowable percentages of the more expensive components.

Some sausages have dropped in meat content, bulked out with rusk and inferior parts of the animal: hamburgers, originally made with good-quality minced steak, have in some cases been degraded into 'burgers' with as much as 40 per cent non-meat ingredients; ham on the bone has largely given way to vacuum-packed re-moulded scraps of pig-meat; some fish fingers have dropped in fish content; dairy products are being imitated by the use of sophisticated technology and non-dairy ingredients; butter is mixed with vegetable fats to create a new spreading fat; skimmed milk or buttermilk and vegetable fat are being marketed as a substitute for cream.

These examples are by no means representative of all foods of their kind, and no one would suggest that in future butter, cream or sausages will have disappeared in their well-known forms for ever. What they do indicate, though, is that there are some manufacturers who are prepared to produce foods the only criterion for which is cost, and that there are consumers prepared to purchase them. The justification is that people need cheap food and are getting good value. The experience of high-quality food is a luxury they do not want, the majority selecting what they habitually buy at the most competitive price.

Far too many manufacturers look no further than considerations of cost-effectiveness, the superficial appeal of novelty and technological efficiency. They have chosen to ignore the traditional art of cooking. Manufactured products are rarely determined by ideas from chefs, but more often by what the food scientists can create or what can be made in their existing machinery, much of which may be old and inefficient. This is inimical to the production of aesthetically good food. The emphasis is on economy of ingredients and production at the lowest possible price, commensurate with safety and nutritional adequacy.

To ignore the role of the chef, or culinary specialist, is the equivalent of asking a decorator to produce a landscape. The outstanding cooks of each new generation are continuing a creative activity, borrowing from the accumulated experience of generations before them, and translating it into something which gives pleasure and excitement to their own generation, as well as inspiring anyone who eats or cooks for their own pleasure. Although in this country we have no 'great tradition' of cuisine, we have always had an awareness of good food, even if formerly only the rich or the upper classes could afford to learn this discrimination. An appreciation of food is still an essential part of British culture.

There is no Machiavellian formula to make us eat something we do not wish to eat, but there is a strategy based on a simple truth. Most of us are surprisingly unobservant, particularly if we continually buy the same things. The fact is, familiar products have changed over the years. Some have improved, but many have gone downhill. Does it have to be like this? How can you put into food production the high ideals of good cooking? What does it entail? What compromises do you have to make in the move from kitchen to production line?

Summer Pudding

Let us suppose, for a moment, that you are a substantial manufacturer of high-quality products, specializing in desserts. You have a wide range of products which sell successfully in the supermarkets of a major national retailer. These are priced higher than those of your competitors, but customers appreciate the standard of ingredients and care in manufacture, and are prepared to pay for that standard. You have invested wisely in a modern plant with a caring workforce and skilled quality-controllers. You have a development team of chefs and technologists and marketing people, who work in conjunction with an equivalent team from major retailers.

One of the major retailers whom you regularly supply decides to launch a new dessert that will fit in nicely with their more established ranges. A classic English dish has been chosen, as traditional dishes of this kind have sold well. It is not over-rich, in line with customer demands for 'healthier' food, and it is fruit-based, another plus, given nutritional advice to eat more fruit and vegetables. People used to make it at home, but with so many instant desserts like fruit yoghurts, ice-creams and gateaux, they have stopped bothering over much with puddings. There is a gap in the market for a new one.

The retailer comes to your offices and presents his project. The new product is to be Summer Pudding, a fruit dessert that has been revived successfully by top restaurants, but has been largely forgotten by town-dwellers. This pudding has the dual advantage of being a popular recipe in British traditional cooking for some, and an intriguing novelty for others. The risk factor is not too high, for a food will usually succeed if it has cultural roots, and as a manufacturer you will prefer to follow trends. A major ice-cream company has translated the idea into an ice-cream version which is very popular. The market seems to be ripe.

The development team gets together. They will probably agree on a definition of Summer Pudding. Apart from the possible addition of alcohol in the fruit, and the substitution of brown bread for white, and honey for sugar, there are no variants in this simple recipe. Everyone from chefs to members of Women's Institutes will recognize a Summer Pudding. In case it is not familiar, here is a standard recipe from the *Good Housekeeping Cook Book*.

Ingredients

> 450–500g mixed blackcurrants,
> blackberries, raspberries, redcurrants
> 2 tbsp water
> 150g sugar
> 100–175g white bread, thinly sliced.

Method

1. Wash and pick over the fruits, string the currants and top and tail them. Put the water and sugar in a large saucepan and bring slowly to the boil. Add the fruits and stew them gently until they are soft but still hold their shape.
2. Cut the crusts off the bread and discard them. Line a 900 ml (1 and a half pint) capacity pudding basin with some of the slices, pour in the stewed fruit mixture and cover with the remaining bread.
3. Place a saucer smaller in diameter than the top of the basin on top of the pudding; weight it down and leave overnight. Turn out and serve with whipped cream or egg custard sauce

The first step towards manufacture happens in the experimental kitchen. The chefs, with hotel and restaurant experience, create the best Summer Pudding possible, with every ingredient of the finest quality they can find. When they are satisfied with the proportions of ingredients, the flavour, texture, cutting-quality, heating and timing of the recipe (they will work more precisely than the domestic cook), the finished product is tasted by representatives from marketing, factory production, and the relevant executives from management. After some negotiation, you try to accommodate different tastes and reactions whilst keeping as near to the recipe as you can, and make only slight changes from what you consider to be an ideal recipe.

The next process hinges round 'bulking up', which means working out how to translate making one or two puddings into a continuous production of thousands. You have to find out:

1. if it is feasible using your existing facilities;
2. if you will need any new facilities;
3. if the whole exercise is economically viable.

A series of meetings is held to find the answers. Here is a summary of what might have happened.

Problem number one is the shape. Summer Pudding is traditionally a pudding-basin shape. Can the existing plant in the factory manufacture that shape? No, it cannot. Can it be adapted to make it? Yes, it can. Will moulds be needed? Yes. How much will they cost? £15 each and 15,000 are needed. A capital investment of £225,000 straight away, and the factory might never make another dessert in that shape again. This is rejected. Another solution is proposed, to market the product in aluminium foil basins. More costings, and the pudding basin is looking just feasible.

Now to the bread. How many loaves will be needed for optimum production? Around 15,000 loaves a week. Where will the bread come from and can a supplier be found to make that quantity to the quality required? Where will it be stored? Can the bread be obtained ready-sliced with the required precision? A local baker is found who is prepared to expand his production and take on extra staff to meet requirements. On the basis of a guaranteed order, a good price is negotiated.

Can fresh fruit be brought in and from where? Does the factory have the facilities to store, handle and prepare it? The answer is no. An outside supplier has to be found who will provide the fruit mixture to a specification. Can it be delivered in two-litre bags to be opened and disposed of on site? The fruit supplier might grumble at the price offered, but a large order is involved. Prices are agreed.

Now for the cooking process. The first problem is how to transfer the fruit mixture into the aluminium basins lined with bread. This is just one of the various processes on the production line which must be precisely worked out. The whole operation must be timed to a split second. Trials are held in the factory to work out the best formula for production. As other products are being made, each time a trial is undertaken it ties up machinery and loses money. Answers must be found quickly. The production planner makes a timetable of when the Summer Pudding will be made, whether it will be a continuous run or several runs during the week.

After all these meetings and detailed discussions, everything is looking good. The chefs are pleased, because they have kept to their original recipe. Everyone else is pleased because solutions have been found which make practical and economic sense. The company will expect to make an adequate profit (around one-fifth of the price) on the pudding, leaving enough for the retailer.

The big day arrives when your client arrives with his team. They like your version of Summer Pudding, and think it will prove

11.3 The story of a summer pudding

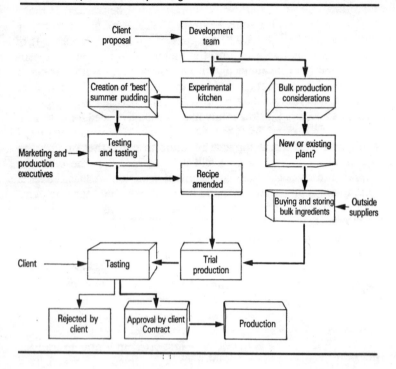

popular. A final go-ahead has not yet been given but everyone is hopeful.

This is a hypothetical case, but it is based on a real situation. In the event, our manufacturer, in spite of all his care, did not receive the contract. Another manufacturer was prepared to compromise on the shape and classic ingredients of the pudding and could make it far more cheaply. He gained the contract, but in this case the public was not to be deceived. The product did not sell and was withdrawn after a few months. Was this perhaps an early indication that we are beginning to opt for better food?

Growing awareness

Good retailers must be highly sensitive to these straws in the wind. Our growing awareness of what good food should be is forcing major retailers to respond quickly to the market. Behind the scenes, food products are constantly changing, and the indications are that these changes involve upgrading.

One retailer, Marks & Spencer, has been in the forefront of the campaign to revolutionize food taste. Although not all their products are entirely satisfactory – as they would be the first to admit – their best is as yet unequalled. They were the first to recognize two fundamental principles of food production: first, that every single ingredient, even down to salt, pepper and sugar, must be the best of its kind and constantly monitored; secondly, that cooking is an art, and should be respected as such. It is common practice for development staff to visit top restaurants all over Britain and abroad to determine what makes certain dishes authentic and special, in order to reproduce them in their experimental kitchens.

There are few go-ahead manufacturers who would dispute that they have a lot to learn from the best chefs, and there are signs, at least in some areas, that the stranglehold exerted by food technologists on the quality of food could be on the wane. Nonetheless, there has also been a reluctance on the part of top chefs to have anything to do with what most of us obtain from supermarket shelves. If manufacturers are edging their way towards an understanding of culinary tradition, then chefs, too, should appreciate the technological and economic constraints of manufactured foods. The cross-fertilization of chef and manufacturer is taken for granted in France, and it could well be more widely copied in Britain.

The tendency towards the cheap and mundane is not restricted to manufactured products. Fresh food has also suffered from these dual standards. Anyone who grows their own fruit or vegetables will be aware of the enormous difference in flavour compared with the beautiful-looking but disappointing plastic-wrapped specimens in a supermarket. In the development of products, flavour is just one of the many factors taken into account. Appearance, resistance to disease and high yield are others. Appearance and keeping-quality may dominate for strawberries grown for the table, but flavour comes top of the list for those grown for jam.

Meat, too, has suffered, particularly beef and chicken. We might dislike the idea of intensive rearing and producing premature weight-gain, but even if these practices are carried out as humanely and efficiently as possible, the quality and character of meat will be predetermined. It is generally accepted in the meat trade that allowing an animal to gain as much weight as possible in the shortest time has affected flavour. Accelerated growth means bland meat for, above all, the development of a mature taste needs time – the older the animal at slaughter, the better it will be. This applies equally to battery chickens, reared for slaughtering at the tender age of twelve weeks.

There are two more candidates for blandness resulting from farming methods: fish and game. Concentrating on breed-selection and manufactured feeds with a high nutrient density, given at precise intervals within a controlled environment, may make economic sense, but those familiar with the taste of wild trout and salmon, venison or game birds, are now fearing another food devaluation.

Top restaurants, quality butchers and fishmongers are aware of this situation, and are prepared to seek out small specialist suppliers, paying a high price in order to obtain quality foods. Some farmers and market-gardeners are rediscovering neglected breeds and varieties, and accepting that they will need more time and care to produce them than the ones that are commercially successful.

The decline in the quality of food need not be inevitable and there are some hopeful signs. There are pressures within the EEC to take 20 per cent of land away from cereal production. If more land becomes available for cattle, it could become economically attractive to return to more extensive systems of rearing, where animals are given the proper time to mature. Fresh fruit and vegetables have been allocated more space in supermarkets and some growers are now prepared to take greater risks in producing the more temperamental, less abundant but more flavourful varieties.

Food manufacturers and retailers then, under pressure from shareholders and consumers, have striven to keep food cheap with the consequent reduction in aesthetic quality. This situation is likely to change only if consumers are prepared to raise their demands for better food.

Really good-quality food is expensive (our European neighbours are accustomed to paying far higher prices) but if enough people are prepared to forego other items in the annual budget in order to eat well, and recent surveys show that, at least outside the home, expenditure on food is rising, then eventually the cost could come down. No one can forecast which category will eventually gain the ascendancy, the good or the indifferent, but if there is an awareness of such a division and why it exists, we might be able to halt the further degradation of our food and encourage those who are trying to lift it from the doldrums.

Manufacturers and retailers must be prepared to play their part. If the strait-jacket of market competition allied to a shortage of consumer cash have driven food-quality downwards, it is possible that more adventurous investment at this time could reap rich dividends, not only for the shareholders but for all who care about good food.

12 Practical Nutrition

*How you can help yourself to a better diet. Healthy
eating messages are redundant when you know what
you are doing*

Lis Leigh

Individuals are not in the habit of thinking consciously about the
quantity of food they eat or the effects it has. A small portion for
one person is large for another. Some people will automatically
interchange foods so that meals are alternately lighter and heavier,
varying the proportion of cooked and uncooked ingredients and
using a wide range of raw materials. Others will find sufficient
variation in substituting baked beans for chips!

The energy content of meals and snacks is not normally taken
into account by the individual. Largely ignored too is the 'ideal'
daily total of energy, to be taken in as food, that is about right for
height, weight and lifestyle. However, most of us do take note of
what the bathroom scales say!

Energy

Energy is *taken in* as food and drink and *given out* whilst maintaining
the functions of the body and carrying out activity. There are
certain components of foods that are essential for health. These are
the nutrients: protein, fat, carbohydrates, vitamins and minerals.

Vitamins and minerals do not provide us with energy, but protein, fat and carbohydrates do. Water (or liquid) is also essential for
health, although not usually considered a 'nutrient'. Each of us
needs about two pints of liquid every day.

Most foods contain a mixture of nutrients (for example a slice of bread will contain protein, carbohydrate, fat, and some vitamins and minerals) and will vary in the energy they provide. Even when a person is completely at rest, energy is still needed to maintain the body's internal organs – to keep the heart beating and the body temperature at around 37 °C, to enable the liver and kidneys to function, and to fuel the brain.

The traditional way of measuring energy was in terms of Calories (kilocalories) – and this is the way most of us still think of it – although kilojoules are now also used. Those who have ever gone on a diet will be familiar with the business of adding up the daily Calories. But how many Calories do we *really need* each day?

That question is tricky, because every individual has different energy requirements, which vary with age, sex, and the amount, intensity and duration of activity. We all know people who can eat like a horse and remain slim, and others who appear not to consume much at all, but are plump.

The DHSS has established a guide which indicates how much energy different *groups* of people need to take in as food and drink each day. These daily Calorie recommendations are not intended for *individuals*, and can only serve as a rough guide. Some people may need a little more and some a little less than the levels set. The DHSS also gives recommendations for daily amounts of nutrients. The levels for these are designed to be *greater* than the requirements of most individuals. Table 12.1 shows part of the DHSS table of recommended daily amounts (RDAs) of food energy and nutrients.

These guidelines were set in 1979, and since then, with the development of the science of nutrition and improved analytical techniques and methods of measurement, more has been discovered about requirement for nutrients. As a nation, we have become generally less active, due among other things to continuing urbanization, automation, information technology, increasing car-ownership and use of convenience meals. A lot of the effort has been taken out of living and working, resulting in a decline in energy expenditure. The RDAs are now being revised to take account of these changes and to incorporate the latest scientific findings.

Instead of thinking in terms of the Calorie count of every mouthful of food eaten, start to appreciate the calorific value of your typical daily meals, snacks and alcohol intake. Table 12.2

gives some variations on breakfast, lunch and dinner, and some snacks and alcohol, with approximate Calorie totals. Some details of nutrients are also given.

Table 12.1 Selected RDAs taken from Recommended Daily Amounts of Food Energy and Nutrients for Groups of People in the UK (1979), report by COMA, DHSS, *Report on Health and Social Subjects*, No. 15. Note that RDAs are intended for groups within the population and so to apply them to individual diets is misleading. They are often used as a general guide.

Age range		Occupational category	Energy	
			MJ	kcals.
Boys	12–14		11.0	2640
	15–17		12.0	2880
Girls	12–14		9.0	2150
	15–17		9.0	2150
Men	18–34	Sedentary	10.5	2510
		Moderately active	12.0	2900
		Very active	14.0	3350
	35–64	Sedentary	10.0	2400
		Moderately active	11.5	2750
		Very active	14.0	3350
	65–74	Assuming a sedentary life	10.0	2400
Women	18–54	Most occupations	9.0	2150
		Very active	10.5	2500
	55–74	Assuming a sedentary life	8.0	1900

Table 12.2 Menus, Snacks and Alcohol with approximate values. Nutritional analysis based on data from A A Paul and D A T Southgate (1979), McCance and Widdowson's, *The Composition of Foods*, 4th rev. ed., HMSO, London.

FOOD	Handy measure	Weight (g)	Energy (kcals.)	Protein (g)	Sugars (g)	Starch and Dextrins (g)	Sat. fatty acids (g)	Poly-unsaturated Fatty Acids (PUFA) (g)
Breakfast 1								
Fruit juice (unsweetened)	1 medium glass	200						
Cereal (cornflakes)	Average serving	37						
Whole milk (for cereal and tea)		280						
Toast (brown)	2 large slices	90						
Butter	2 tsp.	10						
Marmalade	2 tsp.	20						
			711	21.4	39.8	65.0	11.7	1.6

Rounding up of figures to nearest whole number is advised.

Table 12.2 (cont.)

FOOD	Handy measure	Weight (g)	Energy (kcals.)	Protein (g)	Sugars (g)	Starch and Dextrins (g)	Sat. fatty acids (g)	PUFA (g)
Breakfast 2								
Grapefruit segments (tinned NAS*)	Average portion	110						
Bacon (back, lean & fat, grilled)	2 rashers	44						
Egg (fried)	1	50						
Sausage (beef, fried)	1	47						
Toast (white)	2 medium slices	60						
Butter	2 tsp.	10						
Marmalade	2 tsp.	20						
Whole milk (for coffee)	2 tsp.	40						
			778.0	32.0	33.9	35.7	32.0	4.6

* NAS No added sugar

FOOD	Handy measure	Weight (g)	Energy (kcals.)	Protein (g)	Sugars (g)	Starch and Dextrins (g)	Sat. fatty acids (g)	PUFA (g)
Breakfast 3								
Muesli	Average	70						
Semi-skimmed milk (for cereal and tea)		280						
Toast (wholemeal)	2 large slices	100						
Honey	Average	15						
Banana	1 small	100						
Margarine (soft vegetable oils only)	2 tsp.	10						
			809.0	22.1	62.3	70.7	6.9	5.5
Breakfast 4								
Toast (brown)	1 large slice	45						
Butter	1 tsp.	5						
Marmalade	2 tsp.	20						
Whole milk (for coffee)	Average	40						
			165.0	5.4	16.6	18.0	3.6	0.6

Table 12.2 (cont.)

FOOD	Handy measure	Weight (g)	Energy (kcals.)	Protein (g)	Sugars (g)	Starch and Dextrins (g)	Sat. fatty acids (g)	PUFA (g)
Lunch 1								
Tomato soup	1 large bowl	300						
Steak and kidney pie	Average	215						
Mashed potato (boiled plus 5g butter)	Average	150						
Peas (canned, processed)	Average	80						
Beer	1 pint	565						
Cheese (Stilton)	small piece	30						
(Cheddar)	small piece	30						
Butter	2 tsp.	10						
Oatcakes	4	24						
			1720	49.4	2.34	215.3	41.7	7.0
Lunch 2								
Bread (wholemeal)	2 large slices	100						
Margarine	2 tsp.	10						
Ham (boiled, lean and fat)	2 slices	56						
Salad, Tomato		35						
Salad, Cucumber		20						
Salad, Lettuce		10						
Fruit juice	1 average glass	200						
Apple	1 large	150						
Orange	1 medium	165						
Whole milk (for tea)		20						
			621	25	37	40	8	4

Lunch 3

Baked potato + skin	1 average	174					
Quiche Lorraine	Medium piece	200					
Tomato	1 small	70					
Cucumber	Average	30					
Lettuce	Average	33					
French dressing	1 tbs.	14					
Fruit yogurt	1 pot	142					
		1154	51	24	77	27	6

Lunch 4

Roast beef (sirloin)	Average	95					
Yorkshire pud.	Average	30					
Roast potato	Average	129					
Cabbage	Average	60					
Beans (runner)	Average	100					
Apple pie	⅙ of 9″ pie	160					
Custard	4 tbs.	80					
(made with powder)							
Whole milk (for tea)		20					
		1106	37	27	48	32	7

Table 12.2 (cont.)

FOOD	Handy measure	Weight (g)	Energy (kcals.)	Protein (g)	Sugars (g)	Starch and Dextrins (g)	Sat. fatty acids (g)	PUFA (g)
Lunch 5								
Butter	Average	5						
Smoked salmon	Average	80						
Bread (wholemeal)	1 large slice	50						
Rack of lamb	Average	110						
Potatoes (boiled)	Average	120						
French beans	Average	100						
Leeks	Average	60						
Cheese sauce	2 tbs.	38						
Fruit salad								
– Apple		50						
– Orange		50						
– Banana		40						
– Grape		20						
Cream (double)	1 tbs.	15						
Cheese, Cheddar		50						
Cheese, Stilton		30						
Cheese, Camembert		30						
Oatcakes	4	24						
Cream (single for coffee)	1 tbs.	15						
Butter	2 tsp.	10						
			1522	94	28	62	48	6

FOOD	Handy measure	Weight (g)	Energy (kcals.)	Protein (g)	Sugars (g)	Starch and Dextrins (g)	Sat. fatty acids (g)	PUFA (g)
Dinner 1								
Soup (vegetable)	1 medium plate	250						
Roast chicken (light meat)	Average	118						
Potatoes (boiled)	2 average	120						
Sprouts	Average	111						
Carrots	Average	60						
Trifle	Average	150						
Whole milk (for coffee)	Average	40						
			653.0	46.9	40.4	42.3	7	1.4
Dinner 2					Total carbohydrate		Total fat	
Mutton curry		225						
Mango chutney	2 tbls.	30						
Pakoras/Bhajia		150						
Papadums	2	50						
Raita		100						
Rice (boiled)	large portion	300						
Jellabi (ground rice)	Average	150						
			2273.0	74.7	248.2		115.4	

Table 12.2 (cont.)

FOOD	Handy measure	Weight (g)	Energy (kcals.)	Protein (g)	Sugars (g)	Starch and Dextrins (g)	Sat. fatty acids (g)	PUFA (g)
Dinner 3								
Fish (fried)	Average	150						
Chips	Average	145						
Peas (canned, processed)	Average	80						
Bread (wholemeal)	2 small slices	60						
Butter	2 tsp.	10						
Peaches (canned)	Small tin	227						
Cream (double)	Average	60						
			1445.0	47	65	104	45.2	4.0
Dinner 4								
Prawns	Average	28						
Dressing (thousand islands)	2 tbs.	30						
Lettuce	Average	20						
Steak (rump, fried)	Average	160						
Chips	Average	145						
Tomato	1 small	70						
Mushrooms	Average	25						
Lemon meringue pie	Average	200						
Cream (double) (for gateaux and coffee)	Average	80						
			2027.0	69.7	58.5	98.4	61.9	9.1

FOOD	Handy measure	Weight (g)	Energy (kcals.)	Protein (g)	Sugars (g)	Starch and Dextrins (g)	Sat. fatty acids (g)	PUFA (g)
							Total fat	
Dinner 5								
Special chow mein portion								
Noodles		160						
Peas		17						
Chicken		17						
Pork, lean and fat		12						
Prawns		12						
Oil		10						
			813.0	30.7	0.3	116.0		26.9
Dinner 6								
Mac ¼ pounder	1	160						
Chips	Reg.–med. portion	145						
Mac D coke	Medium	330						
Mac apple pie	⅓ of 9" pie	160						
Ice cream (d)	2 scoops	105						
Mac D coffee		30						
			1596.0	38.6	66.5	122.4	39.1	6.7

Table 12.2 (cont.)

FOOD	Handy measure	Weight (g)	Energy (kcals.)	Protein (g)	Sugars (g)	Starch and Dextrins (g)	Sat. fatty acids (g)	PUFA (g)
Dinner 7								
Coleslaw		75						
Pizza, cheese and tomato	Average	150						
Potato (jacket)	1	174						
			891	19	6	72	8	1
Alcohol								
Spirit	1 std measure	25	55.0	0.1	2.2			
Sherry	1 large glass	60	70.8	1.7	13.0			
Bitter	1 pint	565	180.0	1.1	9.0			
Mild	1 pint	565	141.0	1.1	8.0			
Bottled lager	1 pint	565	164.0	3.9	34.0			
Strong ale	1 pint	565	406.0		15.0			
Dry cider	1 pint	565	203.0		24.0			
Sweet cider	1 pint	565	237.0	1.5	2.0			
Red wine	5 glasses	750	510.0	0.7	19.0			
Rosé wine	5 glasses	750	532.0	1.5	44.0			
Sweet white wine	5 glasses	750	705.0	2.2	10.0			
Sparkling white wine	5 glasses	750	570.0	0.8	4.5			
Dry white wine	5 glasses	750	495.0	0.8	25.5			
Medium white wine	5 glasses	750	562.0					

FOOD	Handy measure	Weight (g)	Energy (kcals.)	Protein (g)	Sugars (g)	Starch and Dextrins (g)	Sat. fatty acids (g)	PUFA (g)
Snacks								
Crisps	1 pkt	25.0	130.0	1.6	0.2	9.8	3.6	Figures not available
Treacle tart	1	60.0	223.0	2.3	20.2	16.6	3.3	1.08
Biscuit	1 Penguin	30.0	157.0	1.7	13.0	7.2	5.0	0.34
Digestive (plain)	1	15.0	70.0	1.5	2.5	5.7	1.3	0.3
Peanuts	small pkt	50.0	240.0	12.1	1.5	23.0	4.61	7.0
Chocolate nut bar	1	62.0	315.0	7.0	34.4 Total carbohydrate		7.5	Figures not available
Fruit cake	1 slice	40.0	142.0	2.0	17.0	6.0	2.3	0.45
Mince pie	1	50.0	217.0	2.1	15.0	16.0	Figures not available	

The tables give a broad picture of the Calorie value of some meals. If you want a more accurate picture of *your* Calorie intake, you will need to keep a log of the food and drink taken in over an average week. Make a note of everything you eat and drink, and do not forget take-aways, snacks, sweets, fruit drinks, meals at other people's houses etc. If you are really serious about monitoring your intake (if you have reason to believe you are considerably over- or underweight), a pocket Calorie counter and some food scales could be useful.

Here is one way in which a 40-year-old, moderately active man might obtain his energy and nutrients from food. According to the RDA table (see Table 12.1), he belongs to a group which requires approximately 2750 kcals. daily. The meals are referred to by their number in Table 12.2.

Meal	Energy (kcals)
Breakfast (1)	711
Lunch (2)	621
Dinner (1)	653
Snacks	
2 choc. biscuits	314
packet of peanuts	240
2 standard spirit measures	110
TOTAL	2649

With this daily intake he would be approaching the energy requirement of 2750 kcals.

A 50-year-old very active woman is our second example. Her daily energy requirements will be approximately 2500 kcals.

Breakfast (4)	165
Lunch (3)	1154
Dinner (7)	891
Wine (1 glass)	85
Snack (1 choc. biscuit)	157
TOTAL	2452

A teenage boy's (12–14 years) daily energy requirement would be around 2640 kcals.

Breakfast (3)	809
Lunch (2)	621
Dinner (1)	653
Snacks 2 semi-sweet biscuits	140
Crisps 1 packet	130
Fruit: 1 apple, 1 orange	300
TOTAL	2653

It is unlikely that anyone would eat exactly the same amount of food, or exercise to the same degree every day, so in practice, most people meet their energy needs over a period of, say, a few days.

Alcohol is often left out of calculations, but it can add appreciably to the daily energy total. (Alcohol provides 7 kcals./g.) One pint of beer will contain about 180 kcals., and a glass of red wine, about 85 kcals. Current guidelines suggest that the weekly alcohol intake should be kept within certain limits, expressed in units. One unit is half a pint of beer, a standard measure of spirits, a medium glass of sherry, or a glass of wine.

The recommendations are:

> For a woman: no more than 14 units of alcohol per week
> For a man: no more than 21 units of alcohol per week.

If you are a male beer-drinker, about 10½ pints of beer per week will take you up to the limit. For a woman wine-drinker, up to 14 glasses of wine per week is the recommended limit. It is also recommended that those who drink should have several alcohol-free days in a week.

Note that dry white wine does not have significantly fewer Calories than dry red wine. Sweet wine has nearly 30 kcals. more per glass than dry wine.

Once you have found your approximate energy intake, you need to find out how it matches up to your energy expenditure. Remember, however, that energy taken in does not just fuel physical activities. Approximately three-quarters of it goes in keeping the body working and nothing else. So the energy obtained by the body from food will nowhere near match the energy spent just on activity.

Few of us normally record every detail of our daily activities. However, for the sake of this dietary investigation, the next step is to take an average week and keep an activity diary, noting duration and intensity if possible. Note especially the changes in your routine at weekends. Here is an example – again, do not expect this diary to have scientific precision!

11.30p.m.–7.30a.m.   Asleep.

7.30a.m.   Get up, wash and get dressed, make breakfast, eat it, wash up.

8.15a.m.   Walk quarter of a mile to the bus-stop. Run fast for bus for last 50 yds. Sit down for 20 minutes.

9.00a.m.   Arrive at work, walk up two flights of stairs, go to office. Sit down working at desk.

12.30p.m.   10-minute walk to wine bar. Stand for half an hour. Walk round the shops for half an hour. Return to office, up two flights of stairs.

1.45p.m.   Sit at desk most of the afternoon. Stand and talk to colleague for 10 minutes.

5.30p.m.   Catch bus home. Stand for 10 minutes, sit for 10 minutes. Walk home.

6.10p.m.   Make supper for self and children. Wash up.

7.15p.m.   Read the paper. Play games sitting down. Clear up. Iron two shirts (15 minutes). Watch TV for two hours.

10.00p.m.   Walk dog round the block (10 minutes).

10.30p.m.   Have a bath.

11.00p.m.   Go to bed.

There are different ways of calculating energy spent in physical activities, so you might find variations, but Magnus Pyke in *Success in Nutrition* has worked out a representative range. Table 12.3 gives some of his estimates of energy expenditure.

Energy and thinking

Let's add another activity to this list – thinking! It is often assumed that the effort required in concentrated thought, which can be very fatiguing, must consume a fair number of Calories. The brain normally uses a sugar, glucose, as its fuel source, which is supplied via the blood. A good balanced diet will automatically enable sufficient glucose to reach the brain. Feelings of tiredness after prolonged study are unlikely to result from lack of glucose, and are more likely to be psychological in origin. (This does not mean they

Table 12.3 **Average energy requirements for various activities carried on for one hour**

	kcals.
Sitting	15
Writing	20
Standing (at ease)	20
Typing	16–20
Drawing	40–50
Dressing	33
Washing dishes	50–84
Washing clothes	124–214
Polishing	174
Ironing	59
Sewing	55
Sweeping floors	84–110
Sawing wood	420
House painting	145–160
Dusting	110
Walking	130–240
Walking upstairs	1000
Fast walking	565
Running	600–1000
Cycling	180–600
Swimming	200–700
Sprinting	1240

Note: These figures do not include an allowance for the energy expended in maintaining the basal metabolic rate (BMR) during the activity.

are not real!) Only in exceptional circumstances – for example, in poorly controlled diabetics – will feelings of weariness and confusion occur that are directly attributable to a fall in the amount of glucose available to the brain.

Nutrients

The energy you take in and the energy you expend is only part of the nutritional picture. Let us now turn to the range of nutrients necessary for health. Nutritionally, it is far better to have some variety in your diet, but this does not mean constant change. Even within a range of traditional, non-exotic meals, you can obtain the right spread of all the nutrients – fat, carbohydrates, protein, vitamins and minerals – in the appropriate amounts. Knowing which foods contain which nutrients will allow you to achieve a balanced and varied diet.

Fat

Fats are made from fatty acids (*see* Chapter 4). There are two main types of fatty acids: saturated and unsaturated (which includes mono- and polyunsaturated). Both types provide 9 kcals. of energy per gram. To complicate matters, most foods contain a mixture of saturated and unsaturated fatty acids in differing proportions. Fat is obtained from a whole range of foods: cooking oils and fats, cakes, biscuits, chocolate, dairy products and meats.

A diet high in fat, particularly saturated fat, has been linked to the development of coronary heart disease (*see* Chapter 5). Recent recommendations have advised us to obtain about one-third of our energy from fat, and this means that many people could benefit from reducing their total intake of fat, particularly their intake of saturated fat.

The main sources of saturated fatty acids in most UK diets are:

> Butter
> Lard
> Hard margarines
> Fat on meat
> Some meat products
> Milk and cheese

In most UK diets, the main sources of unsaturated fatty acids are:

> Vegetable oils
> Soft margarines
> Fish
> Poultry

Lean meat
Some cereals
Cereal products

If you think you have a high-fat intake (your 7-day diary will indicate whether or not you frequently eat large amounts of foods containing fat), there are three ways you could reduce the fat in your diet. You can:

1. Decrease the number of times you eat high-fat foods.
2. Eat smaller portions of high-fat foods.
3. Try lower-fat alternatives now and again.

Bearing in mind that fat provides energy, you will notice that by cutting down your fat intake you will also be cutting back on your energy intake. This is all very well if you wish to lose weight, but if you wish to keep your weight as it is you need to replace the lost energy from other sources. Expert medical opinion suggests that the best way to do this is to increase your intake of carbohydrate foods, especially those rich in 'dietary fibre' – such as bread, potatoes, pasta and rice.

It must be stressed that foods containing fats are not bad for you. We all need some fat in our diets, but we should try to gauge how much fat we need.

Carbohydrates
Sugars and starches are both carbohydrates, and provide the same amount of energy per gram, about 4 kcals.

Sugars are naturally present in fruits, fruit juices, vegetables and milk. They also occur in some processed foods, sweets and drinks. *The body does not differentiate between sugars naturally present and sugars added during the processing of manufactured food.*

Starches are found in bread and flour products, cereals, pasta, rice and some vegetables.

Fibre is largely a mixture of special types of carbohydrates that are not digested. Some fibre in our diets is necessary for the efficient functioning of the bowel. Foods rich in fibre include wholemeal and brown bread, wholegrain cereals, fruit and vegetables.

Proteins
Proteins are needed for the growth and repair of the body, but they can also be used to provide energy. Good sources of protein in the diet include meat, fish, eggs, cheese, milk, poultry and pulses (peas, beans and lentils).

Vitamins and minerals
These are only required in very small amounts, but they are essential for a healthy body. They occur in a range of foods in differing amounts, another important reason for a varied daily diet.

Vitamin and mineral supplements If a person is eating a balanced diet which contains a variety of foods, including fruits and vegetables, vitamin and mineral supplements will not usually be necessary. Some groups in the population might require supplements, for example, pregnant women or people who are eating a poor diet. On the whole, however, there is no virtue in taking vitamins and minerals in (usually expensive) pill form, notwithstanding the heavy promotion these products are given in some magazines and health-food shops.

Fluid
It is important to have an adequate intake of fluid each day – about 6 to 8 glasses of water or its equivalent in tea, coffee or fruit juice etc. To regard alcohol as the principal fluid source is not advisable! (*See* page 181.)

To summarize, there are three simple rules to ensure a healthy diet.

1. Eat a variety of foods but not too much.
2. About a third of your energy should come from fat.
3. Take plenty of fluid but go easy on the alcohol.

Ideal weight

Gaining or losing weight is the most obvious effect of getting the energy balance wrong. Some people like to be on the plump side, others prefer the lean and hungry look. But whatever you feel about your weight, if it stays at a more or less constant level, the chances are your energy *intake* from food and drink is sufficient to meet your energy *output*. If, over a period of time, you take in *more* energy than you need, you will put on weight. If your energy intake is consistently *less* than you require, you will lose weight. Few people eat the same amount of food or exercise to the same extent every day, so in practice it is important to balance your energy over a few days.

12.1 Weight for height chart

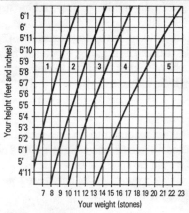

Your height (feet and inches)

6'1
6'
5'11
5'10
5'9
5'8
5'7
5'6
5'5
5'4
5'3
5'2
5'1
5'
4'11

7 8 9 10 11 12 13 14 15 16 17 18 19 20 21 22 23
Your weight (stones)

1	Underweight. Are you eating enough?
2	OK. This is the desirable weight range for health
3	Overweight. Your health could suffer - don't get any fatter!
4	Fat. It's important for you to lose weight
5	Very fat. This is severe and treatment is urgently required

Source: Joint Advisory Committee on Nutrition Education (1985), 'Eating for a Healthier Heart', British Nutrition Foundation/Health Education Council, London

Take a straight line up from your weight (without clothes) and a line across from your height (without shoes). Where the two lines meet tells you how your weight rates. If you are "overweight", "fat" or "very fat", you can lose weight by reducing fat intake. But in this case make sure you don't replace the fat with other foods! Cutting down on sugar and alcohol will also help you to lose weight and be more healthy.

Be prepared to lose weight gradually. Using up body fat takes time. Diets that make you lose weight very quickly are not usually very effective because most of the weight you lose is water rather than body fat and this can return as quickly as it was lost.

Taking some regular exercise will also help. But don't overdo it. If you're not used to exercise, start with brisk walking before moving on to exercises like swimming, cycling or jogging.

A lower fat diet combined with moderate regular exercise is a healthy way to slim. It is also training your body to a new and healthier way to live. Once you've reached your target weight you will be able to increase your food intake. But don't go back to fatty foods. Instead step up the healthier starchy carbohydrate foods with fibre in them such as potatoes, bread, breakfast cereals, rice and pasta including wholegrain varieties.

Medical opinion has concluded that the most important thing in keeping healthy is to keep your weight within the normal range for your height. Figure 12.1 below will help you to gauge whether you are within the correct weight range for your height.

If you are in the overweight, fat or very fat category you should lose weight by:

1. Reducing your energy intake, that is, eat less! Choose a reduced-Calorie diet which contains a variety of foods and adequate amounts of nutrients. A sensible reducing diet will allow weight to be lost gradually while eating habits are adjusted.
2. Increase your energy output, that is, take more exercise. Try walking whenever possible rather than going by car or bus. Try walking up stairs instead of taking the lift. Do not expect dramatic results, but every little helps and you will feel better (eventually).

Here is a sample diet for someone accustomed to an energy intake of 2500 kcals. which has resulted in an excess-weight gain. The sensible way to start reducing would be to set a target of around 1500 kcals. a day. This should give a weight loss of between 1 and 2 lb (approximately 500 g to 1 kg) a week.

BREAKFAST	ENERGY: Calories
Fruit juice, 1 glass	66
Toast, wholemeal, 1 slice	108
Margarine	73
Marmalade	52
LUNCH	
Ham (2 medium slices)	150
Salad: tomatoes, cucumber, lettuce	10
Margarine	73
Bread (2 slices, wholemeal)	216
Yoghurt (fruit)	115
DINNER	
Roast beef (95 g)	270
Potatoes (boiled 120 g)	96

French beans (100 g)	7
Fruit salad (no sugar added)	82
Half-pint daily allowance of semi-skimmed milk for tea/coffee	140
TOTAL	1458

If you are underweight according to Figure 12.1, try to increase your energy intake. Try eating larger portions and introduce a couple of snacks during the day in addition to meals. You should still take some exercise.

Very low calorie diets (VLCDs)

A recent arrival in the slimming market has been very low calorie diets (VLCDs). The term is generally used to apply to a diet which reduces the daily food-energy intake to below 600 kcals. for several consecutive days or weeks. Usually these dietary preparations, which can come in the form of powders or bars, achieve the low-Calorie intake by totally replacing normal meals. The formulation must supply adequate amounts of all nutrients.

Ideally, slimmers only want to lose fat from their bodies, but protein and minerals can also be lost when energy intake is restricted. The more restricted the diet, the greater the loss of these body components and it may be that these losses could be too great.

A report by a Government Advisory Committee in 1987 made the following recommendations to the general public.

For anyone wishing to lose weight, it is suggested that they should first try to reduce their food-energy intake along conventional lines, that is via a reduced Calorie diet. The use of VLCDs is not recommended as a method of weight reduction for the mildly obese or plump individuals, or for those wishing to lose weight for cosmetic reasons.

People considering the use of VLCDs are strongly advised to check with their doctor first, to ensure that this method is suitable for them. The use of VLCDs as a sole source of nourishment should not exceed the period recommended by the manufacturer, and if the VLCD regime is followed for longer than a few weeks medical supervision is required. VLCDs are *not* suitable for children, pregnant and breast-feeding women and the elderly.

Other Diets

Many books have been written advocating the ideal diet for slimmers, each rivalling the other in miraculous weight loss. The main points to remember are that any diet should be well-balanced and include a variety of foods. If a diet is based on a single food (often a fruit), or recommends a small number of foods as having particular properties, there is a strong possibility that such a diet will be unbalanced, and hence have harmful consequences over a long period.

A good reducing diet needs time. If you plan to lose weight, do not decide on a drastic reduction but start a month or so before you wish to reach your goal. A steady weight loss of 1–2 lb (500 g–1 kg) per week is a realistic goal.

Remember above all, that:

A healthy diet is a well-balanced one which will keep your weight within the right range for your height.

Shopping

Having a week's menu of food to follow, together with specified quantities, to give the right spread of nutrients and keep obesity at bay seems appealing. But in reality it does not make nutritional sense because requirements, lifestyles and food preferences are different for each individual. However, let us assume that you buy most foods for the week in one trip. The typical amounts of some major food groups consumed by a family of four (two adults, two children) in a week, might look like the shopping basket in Figure 12.2. These amounts do not include alcohol or food eaten outside the home, on average 3.7 meals per person per week.

Apart from the shopping list shown in Figure 12.2 other common sources of particular nutrients are:

Protein: nuts, pulses (peas, beans and lentils), cereals.

Calcium: bones in canned sardines and salmon, eggs, nuts.

12.2 The weekly shop

Figures based on a family of two adults and two children.

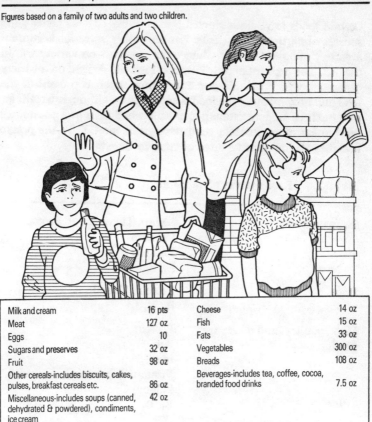

Milk and cream	16 pts	Cheese	14 oz
Meat	127 oz	Fish	15 oz
Eggs	10	Fats	33 oz
Sugars and preserves	32 oz	Vegetables	300 oz
Fruit	98 oz	Breads	108 oz
Other cereals-includes biscuits, cakes, pulses, breakfast cereals etc.	86 oz	Beverages-includes tea, coffee, cocoa, branded food drinks	7.5 oz
Miscellaneous-includes soups (canned, dehydrated & powdered), condiments, ice cream	42 oz		

Data does not include alcoholic drinks or food eaten outside the home. On average 3.7 meals per person per week are eaten outside the home.

NB This shopping basket illustrates the *amounts* of some major foods typically eaten by a family of four in the course of a week. Within these groups the *types* of foods chosen will vary, e.g. lower fat milks may be chosen in preference to whole milk, wholemeal bread may be chosen in preference to white bread. The choice is a matter for the individual. In making the choice, it is important for the individual to consider the general guidelines pertaining to diet and the sections dealing with energy and nutrients, particularly those focusing on fat and carbohydrates.

Source: Adapted from MAFF (1985) Annual Report of the National Food Survey Committee, Household Food Consumption and Expenditure, *HMSO, London. The Biscuit, Cake, Chocolate and Confectionery Alliance (1987),* Annual Review, *BCCCA, London.*

Vitamin D: also produced by the action of sunlight on the skin.

Certain foods have been singled out in Table 12.4 as being good sources of particular nutrients. But remember, most foods contain a variety of others as well – hence the emphasis on variety within the diet. The amount of nutrients obtained will depend on a variety of factors, which include principally how much is present in the food and how much of the food is eaten. Thus, although weight for weight there is more vitamin C in an orange than in a potato, we tend to eat more potatoes than oranges in the UK, so the potato becomes an important source of vitamin C.

Table 12.4 **Food sources of nutrients**

Dairy products	Sugars (lactose), Fat, Protein Calcium Vitamin A B_1, B_2
Eggs	Protein, Vitamin A B_1, B_2
Meat, poultry, and meat products	Protein Fat Iron Vitamin A (especially liver and kidney) B_1, B_2
Fish	Protein Fat (esp. in fatty fish) Vitamin A (esp. fish liver oils) Vitamin D (esp. fatty fish)
Fats/Oils	Fat Vitamin A (butter & margarine) Vitamin D (margarine & butter)
Sugars, preserves (jam, marmalade) & confectionary	Sugar
Cakes, biscuits	Starch, sugars, fat B vitamins

Bread, cereals	Sugars/starch, Dietary fibre Protein, Iron, Calcium Vitamins B_1, B_2
Potatoes	Starch, Protein, Iron Range of vitamins and minerals Vitamin C
Fruits	Sugars, Range of vitamins and minerals, Vitamin C Dietary fibre
Vegetables	Dietary fibre Iron, Calcium (esp. green veg.) Vitamin A (dark green & yellow) Range of vitamins and minerals

To summarize. Eat every day:

Good helpings of: bread, potatoes, cereals, fruit and vegetables.

Choose from: lean meats, poultry, fish; cheese, eggs or pulses.

Have some: milk, cheese, yoghurt.

Have small amounts of: oils and fats (butter, margarine, cooking oils and fats)

Have occasionally: sweets, biscuits, cakes, fizzy drinks, crisps.

Causes for concern

Fashions, by their very nature, come and go, and this is just as true of food as it is of fashion. 'Healthy eating' is now fashionable – and food-scares make headlines.

For the non-specialist member of the public who has neither the qualifications nor the time to study research documents, the truth behind food-scares is hard to establish. For example, reason may tell you that the minute amount of additives consumed in a year is unlikely to be harmful, but fashion says you should reject them all out of hand. How much attention should the busy shopper give to well-publicized food-scares? What lies behind them? Does it mean avoiding certain foods in pursuit of health?

Cholesterol (see also Chapter 5)
Will the cholesterol naturally present in foods such as meat, eggs, seafood and fish, lead to a heart attack?
At one time, it was considered advisable to eat no more than three eggs a week. Further research on body cholesterol has shown that this advice was over-cautious. Only a very high intake of dietary cholesterol will affect body cholesterol. Unless medically advised to the contrary, you do not need to exclude products containing cholesterol from the shopping basket, for many will contain valuable nutrients.

Snacks
Should children be banned from consuming certain manufactured foods?
Quite rightly, parents are anxious to provide their children with foods that will allow them to grow healthily. Much propaganda has been aimed at rules to be followed by parents and schools. Conflicting messages are put out by the food industry, journalists and some dietitians. It is difficult for a parent to make a decision when confronted by a child who wants something popularly considered 'bad'. The most vociferous campaigns have been waged against sugary foods and savoury snacks: crisps, bottled drinks, sweets and chocolates. Where should we draw the line?

As long as the main diet is varied, products which children find pleasurable and fun to eat are all right within reason. Care should be taken to make sure such foods are not the basis of the daily diet, for no single food contains all the nutrients that children (or adults) need.

Tooth decay (*Dental caries*) (*see also* page 131)
How often should children eat sweets?
Sugars and some other foods and drinks are capable of causing tooth decay. This does not mean that children have to stop eating them, as many of these foods are useful sources of energy and other nutrients, but it is sensible to limit the number of times they are eaten. No one should eat and drink more than five times a day, including snacks and sugary drinks. And everyone should clean their teeth at least twice a day, morning and night.

Supplements, intelligence and good behaviour (*see also* Chapter 5)
'If I eat up all my greens, can I stay up later?'

Recent studies have suggested that a child's basic intelligence and behaviour can be improved by vitamin and mineral supplements. Although these studies started with the assumption that there was some nutritional deficiency in children's present diet, this has not been shown to be so. The studies need to be repeated and it will be some time before we know the truth.

The diets of schoolchildren
Is it true that our schoolchildren are badly nourished?
A report published by the DHSS in April 1986 examined the diets of a representative group of schoolchildren in Britain. The findings showed that on average all the groups of children were taller and heavier than expected. Generally their nutrient intakes were above the RDAs, but some girls had low levels of iron, calcium and riboflavin (vitamin B) and some were taking in less energy than recommended for their age. As has been mentioned previously, RDAs (*see* Table 12.1) are designed for groups, and not individuals. There will always be some people who require more or less than the stated amount, so these findings do not necessarily imply a deficiency. If energy intakes had been seriously low, one would have expected the children to be shorter or lighter for their age. This was not the case, but it is possible that a better balance of energy-giving nutrients might be appropriate for some.

Vegetarianism
Is it healthier to become a vegetarian?
There are about one and a quarter million vegetarians in this country who omit meat from the diet either for reasons of economy, or because they believe it is healthier not to eat animal foods, or because they dislike the idea of slaughtering. Because the lifestyles of vegetarians usually differ in other respects as well as the diet, it is not certain that the apparent health benefits are entirely due to the exclusion of animal products from the diet. On balance, however, it is likely that a properly planned vegetarian diet need not be hazardous and might offer health benefits.

If you are thinking of changing your normal diet by cutting out meat, you will need time to make the adjustment. Eating vegetarian food for one day a week will give you the chance to see if you find the idea attractive, and to get used to changing shopping and cooking habits. You can then gradually increase the meatless days over a period of weeks. Another way is to avoid red meat for a while, then poultry and finally fish. Do not make the mistake of eating your normal diet minus meat and fish. It is important to make good your loss of nutrients, particularly protein, from other sources such as eggs, cheese, nuts and pulses.

If you become a strict vegetarian or vegan, excluding eggs and dairy products, or even if you are a lacto-vegetarian (eating dairy products), you must make sure you are obtaining a full complement of all the amino acids you require (*see* Chapter 4). This can be achieved by combining a cereal and a pulse together, for example, baked beans on toast, bean stew with rice or pasta, hummous and pitta.

Dairy foods provide calcium but, for vegans who exclude them, nuts and leafy vegetables are an alternative source. Meat and liver are the prime providers of iron, so this, too, needs to be watched. If you exclude these foods, wholemeal bread, nuts, and pulses, and dark-green leafy vegetables (spinach, broccoli, spring greens) are alternative sources of iron.

Vitamin B_{12} is the vitamin most likely to be missing from vegetarian diets, as it is found mainly in foods of animal origin. Some fermented foods such as beer and tempeh (soya-bean press cake) contain this vitamin, and some yeast extracts and soya milks are supplemented with B_{12}.

If you have children on a vegetarian diet, apart from observing the principles outlined above, you need to watch that they are taking in enough energy. Vegetarian diets tend to be bulky and so fill up a child more quickly, but although he or she may feel full it does not necessarily mean that the child is getting enough energy. Make sure that children are gaining weight normally, and are eating foods with enough of the required energy and nutrients, such as the carbohydrates in bread, potatoes, rice and pasta together with some fat and enough protein.

Keys to a balanced diet

Adhere to the basic principles of diet, and you will stand the best chance of remaining healthy and feeling well.

1. Eat a variety of foods to ensure that you take in all of the essential nutrients.

2. The total fat content of your diet should provide you with about one-third of your energy.

3. Drink adequate amounts of fluid but go easy on the alcohol.

4. Keep your weight within the right range for your height.

13 How to Survive Food Marketing

See through the tinsel and the hype and do your own thing

David M Conning and Barry D Ricketts

The main functions of the modern food industry are food production and food retailing. The first involves agriculture, horticulture and fishing to produce the raw materials of food, and food manufacture, which is the conversion of basic foodstuffs into the familiar dietary components. Both of these activities involve food processing to varying degrees, culminating in the processes of mixing, cooking and presentation.

Distribution to the point of sale, whereby consumers may acquire the finished product, then takes place. Today, food supermarkets dominate the retail trade, and the function of distribution to these outlets is carried out by manufacturers, by third-party distribution specialists or by the supermarket operators' own fleets. This has become a highly sophisticated activity, often involving global transport with the attendant need to preserve the produce.

The market for food has two characteristics which make it unique. The first is its permanence. Whatever else happens, people must eat and therefore, in modern urbanized society, must buy food. The food industry is thus assured of a market for its wares. But the second characteristic is that this market is almost constant in size in any particular country. The size of the market is directly related to the size of the population. Although the world population is increasing inexorably, that of the developed countries is slightly reducing, which means that individual manufacturers and retailers have to compete with each other for a share of the available business.

This has led to a more intense and complicated marketing environment for food products than exists for almost any other retail sector. No new food product has a hope of even making it to the supermarket shelf, unless accompanied by a huge weight of national advertising expenditure, designed to capture the attention of both the retail trade and the individual purchaser.

Nor does this intensive campaign to seize 'market share' consist simply of advertisements in the press, on posters, or television – although these media tend to dominate in weight of expenditure. 'Below the line activities' – editorial press campaigns, in-store promotions, competitions (often involving coupons on the product package), lavish point-of-sale advertising, product demonstrations, sponsorship, and plain and simple discounting ('money-off' offers) – are all fair game in the frantic struggle for a share of the shoppers' budget.

The odds against success in this highly competitive field are frightening. A majority of all new grocery products introduced into the supermarket trade fail within the first six weeks of their launch. Even more products never make it as far as the supermarket shelf, having been rejected – denied 'listing' in the trade jargon – by the exacting specialist buyers employed by the supermarkets to ensure that every square inch of shelf-space in the store achieves a pre-set profit target.

The cost of developing new food products is phenomenal. It is no good presenting the supermarket buyers with a vague product idea. It must be complete, the production and delivery system installed, running and demonstrably reliable; the advertising concept finalized and the space booked. This will have cost millions in the case of a new product; hundreds of thousands even for the extension to an existing range.

The stakes are high, the rewards, in terms of market or brand leadership, are often short-lived. For if the new product is a success, then competitors will follow it into the market-place with 'Me too' products within a very short space of time, and the all-powerful trade will insist that the manufacturer produces 'own-label' versions of the product. Thus hapless manufacturers find themselves competing not only with the opposition, but with their own production under the customer's label (for which they obviously receive less profit). All this competition takes place against a background of a slow but steady decline in the share of individual income devoted to food expenditure.

The consequences of the intense competition as it exists in Britain are many, often contradictory, and not always welcome to those who feel they have a particular responsibility for consumer welfare. Several factors are involved.

Price

The British like their food to be plentiful and cheap and, until recently, have not worried too much about the quality. Britain has to import 30 to 40 per cent of its food from overseas, increasingly from Europe. This is expensive. There have been great efforts over many years therefore to make the most of what we have. In this country, perhaps more than many others, we have developed ways to make food last longer, while retaining a good appearance and remaining wholesome and safe. The result of those endeavours has been a plentiful supply of cheap food, but often of a quality that does not endear itself to those who seek hedonistic experience from eating.

Presentation and 'claims'

In the unending struggle for a share of a fixed, even marginally declining market, advertising becomes intense. This makes use of all of the avenues available in the media, but also involves the presentation of products in the most attractive ways possible – hence the tremendous upsurge in food packaging experienced in the last twenty years.

It is a natural characteristic of advertisers to emphasize the good points of their products, and to minimize or ignore the less-favourable aspects, and this characteristic is accentuated as competition intensifies. It is also typical of them to latch on to whatever fashions or gimmicks are currently in favour with consumers. This is manifested most clearly in the claims made on behalf of the product by the advertiser. Hence if consumers seem to favour food that is 'fresh' or 'natural' or 'healthy', these words will appear with great frequency in adverts and on packages, even when the nature of the product makes the legitimate use of such

13.1 100% natural with no sugar added!

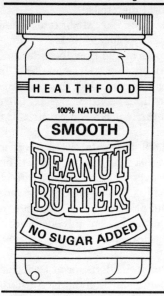

Sugar is not added to this peanut butter – but concentrated apple juice is! This packaging misleads because concentrated apple juice is not natural and is used here on account of its high sugar content. Thus a lot of sugar is added to the product but not in the pure form of sucrose.

words tenuous in the extreme. Margarine, perhaps the epitome of manufactured food, for example, will be described as 'natural' because the original vegetable oil did indeed originate in growing corn or similar seeds.

There are many examples of the way advertisers latch on to contemporary consumer fashions. If they perceive that a sizeable group of consumers has been persuaded to a given viewpoint, that view will be emphasized. Thus the misguided view that sucrose is hazardous, leads so-called 'health food' manufacturers to claim 'sugar free' when they have used grape juice or apple juice, each loaded with sugars (but not sucrose) to sweeten the product; 'no added sugar' when the product is already sweet enough. Similarly 'additive free' appears on products that never contained additives; or 'no preservatives' on products that have a range of other additives. 'No artificial colour' might mean the manufacturer has used a natural colour to artificially colour his product. At least with artificial (i.e. synthesized) colours you know they are made to agreed specifications that govern technical purity, and that they have been fully tested to government requirements. This is not always the case with so-called natural materials.

Advertising may take on a more subtle cloak. Major retailers, for example, have conducted campaigns to educate their consumers on the nutritional value of their products and how to understand the nutritional information printed on their packages. This information nearly always claims or suggests that the particular product is the top of its class for nutritional content, irrespective of whether the individual consumer actually needs those nutrients to that extent.

The published recommended daily amounts (RDAs) of, for example, vitamins are frequently abused in this way. Often one may see that a given product will deliver one-half of the RDA, but not that this might be twice as much as that particular consumer needs. A harmless enough deception, perhaps, if the product is no more expensive than it would otherwise be, but intended, nevertheless, to convey a sense of improved quality that may be spurious.

The consumer enjoys a measure of protection – or at least some recourse – in the form of the Advertising Standards Authority (ASA), set up some twenty-five years ago to take up complaints about misleading advertising with manufacturers and their advertising agencies. Of course, before such a procedure can be effective, the public has to know, or at least suspect, that an advertisement is making spurious or unsupportable claims. However, today's consumer and the organized consumer-representative groups are vigilant, and not slow to exercise the right of complaint.

Perhaps surprisingly, in the light of the intensive competition in food marketing, the ASA feels that the food industry has its house fairly well in order compared with, for instance, the motor trade or electrical appliance manufacturers. Only three cases of misleading claims have been dealt with recently, two of which concerned health claims on behalf of milk products. While these cases were upheld, and the advertising amended or withdrawn, the evidence presented by the defendants in one of the milk examples showed great diligence in seeking medical opinion in the preparation of the advertisement.

The fact remains that while competition is so intense, the temptation to stray over the narrow line between enthusiastic presentation and false claiming is ever-present.

Manufacturer/retailer competition

As the retail sector has become concentrated on fewer companies, these companies wield tremendous power over manufacturers and consumers alike. Unless manufacturers conform to the retailers' demands, they will lose the retail outlets necessary to maintain their market share. The only compromise possible is, as mentioned earlier, in the production of a retailer's 'own brand' or 'own-label' product made by the manufacturer in the image of a product that the manufacturer has already established, but to slightly different standards of quality. The manufacturer is attracted by the potential volume of sales but the upshot is a reduction in choice to the consumer. It may appear the consumer has a choice between two items but there is little to choose between them.

The manufacturer, of necessity, has to adapt production methods to meet the price the retailer is prepared to pay. This may involve marginal changes in the quality and quantity of the raw materials used. Such marginal changes may not be noticeable to the consumer, or may be masked by other ingredients, or indeed may be acceptable. But marginal savings mean a great deal of money when the turnover is very large.

13.2 Pandering to food fashion

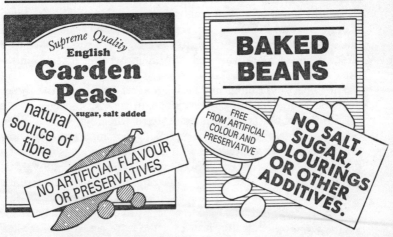

The concentration of power in the hands of fewer retailers also has the potential to restrict consumer choice, in that the retailer will carry only those items that ensure large volume sales and rapid turnover. Less popular items are dropped from the range and the customer can only buy what is available. In practice, this penalty may be more apparent than real for it is itself curtailed by competition among retailers. They pride themselves on their service to the customer, and it is the very expansion of the range of goods carried that may be construed as the cornerstone of this service.

This has had effects which have been very much in the consumer's interest. A number of the major retailers now include specialist departments within their stores, catering for a wider variety of tastes than the mere commodity brands. Whereas a few years ago, we were lucky to find sliced bread in white and wholemeal versions, now, specialized in-store bakeries produce fresh bread products of all kinds, round the clock. The same is often true of coffee and delicatessen products.

Of course, this welcome development is as much a recognition by the retailer that the delicious aroma of fresh bread and coffee, and visually exciting 'deli' displays, can dramatically stimulate sales, but it is welcome none the less. There has also been a tendency for the supermarkets' venture into such specialized areas to educate the tastes of their customers, who then patronize specialist shops which can offer even greater variety and more obscure types of domestic and foreign produce. The delicatessen trade in certain more affluent areas of the country is enjoying a renaissance as a direct result of more educated consumers seeking more sophisticated taste experiences.

The impact of fashions and fads can affect profoundly the choice available to the consumer. The campaign against sausages with a certain fat-content made it difficult, for a while, for some of us to buy a decent banger, although mercifully, common sense has now prevailed, and we are regaled with a full range of 'dogs' in low-fat and good, old-fashioned 'deadly' guise! The campaign against colours and sweeteners made it difficult to buy other than genuine fruit drinks at twice the price and possibly half the satisfaction.

Happily, such fashions tend to be short-lived though they can be very misleading while they last. Taken to extremes, such ill-advised fads are positively dangerous. There have been cases of consumers making themselves ill through over-indulgence in such products as carrot-juice and fibre, under the mistaken impression that a health-benefit would result. So seriously does the A S A take the matter of health-abuse through dieting, that it provides a *British Code of Advertising Practice for Slimming Products*.

Additives and ingredients

As we have seen, the use of additives in manufactured foods has been developed to a high pitch by the advances of food science and technology as applied to industrial production. As we have also seen, where a market potential opens up for goods with reduced additives, the manufacturers are quick to respond by reducing their use. There may be penalties in shorter shelf-life, less attractive products and greater expense, but many consumers are willing to accept those constraints. It remains the case that it is not feasible to remove all additives and still retain a wide choice, but it is possible for the consumer to know what the additives are by using the E system described earlier. Of course this places an onus on the consumer to learn the system and select food accordingly.

The same applies to ingredients. All manufactured food must carry a list of ingredients on the label so that the consumer knows what is in the food being purchased. This might be of crucial importance to some consumers who need to avoid certain ingredients, but is likely to be of little consequence to the vast majority who have no such problems. Nevertheless the information is there if needed.

Packaging

There can be little doubt that the marked advances in food packaging in recent years have revolutionized the purchase of food. The widespread use of plastics has not only transformed food hygiene, but has added considerably to the convenience of the purchase and storage of food. Vacuum packaging and controlled atmosphere packaging have further advanced these benefits. At the same time, the trend towards packaging more and more foods has considerably

13.3 Labelling that helps you choose

Nutrition Information (Amount per 100 grams).

Energy	1978 kJ/471 kcal
Protein	6.3g
Carbohydrate	63g (of which sugars 13g)
Fat	21g (of which saturates 8.3g)
Sodium	0.6g
Fibre	2.9g

This type of label gives you factual information about the product, but you need to know the overall facts about diet and nutrition to decide on a diet that suits you, and whether the product fits into that diet. Reading this book will give you those basic facts.

Source: Government guidelines on good nutrition labelling

increased the scope for messages designed to entice the customer.

Some of these messages are good, providing information the consumer can use; others, as suggested earlier, have been designed to catch the eye and trigger responses in line with contemporary ideas about food. We tend to accept all of these factors as part of life's rich pattern when dealing with the many purchases we have to make in a lifetime. We expect salespeople to accentuate the good points, and we expect advertisers to sail close to the wind.

But when it comes to food, somehow the exaggerated claims are reprehensible and even amoral. This is not just because food and well-being are inextricably linked in our minds. It is also because we have always assumed that the food producers have done all that is required to satisfy our needs. We have come to depend on the fact that good food is always available, plentiful and cheap and have not questioned the wherewithal.

If we want to take a more critical look at what we eat, two things are necessary. First we must have information, and secondly we must know how to use it.

Information

Three sets of information are needed to determine the suitability of food.

1. *The ingredients* It is a legal requirement for most packaged foods and beverages that the contents, including all the components and additives, must be listed on the package in language that we can understand. Many of the materials have cumbersome names, and abbreviations such as E numbers have been tried. The use of E numbers was not an attempt to disguise or obscure but to simplify. Those who really want to know have no difficulty using the system, and it has the added advantage of being standard throughout the EEC.

2. *The freshness* It is important that the food we eat is free of spoilage and possible hazard from contamination. We need to know, therefore, how long the food is likely to last after we have bought it, and under what conditions it needs to be kept to ensure its freshness. The requisite information is incorporated in what is known as 'the shelf life', often expressed as 'best before' dates, with other guidance on the mode of storage. This is often co-ordinated with a simple star system to indicate the type of fridge or freezing compartment that should be used – always supposing the fridge is working properly. Following this information allows the consumer to know how much leeway there is for any particular foodstuff.

3. *Nutrition information* Knowing what is in the food does not always tell us how nutritious it is. For that you need to know about energy, protein, fats, carbohydrates, vitamins and minerals. Thus we need to have nutrition-labelling. The government has issued guidelines on how the nutritional content of foods may be depicted on the packet, or by means of accompanying pamphlets where food is not pre-packaged. The way such information can be conveyed in catering establishments is under consideration.

The guidelines seek to present the information in a factual way and to avoid judgemental statements, such as whether the content of a particular nutrient or component is high or low. This is because only consumers really know the totality of foods they consume and the make-up of individual foods in their diets. This brings us to the second problem.

There is little point in having the information if we do not know how to use it, and few of us know enough about nutrition to be able to work it all out. Even if we could, we get to know our likes and dislikes at a fairly early age after which it is not easy to change and stick to the change.

Although books like this can help those who really want to understand about nutrition, the best time to start is at school or in the home. We all have a responsibility to ensure that our children are better informed about food than we are.

This doesn't mean responding to every new fad that comes along. It does mean learning the basic facts and using them when we make or buy meals.

14 The Future

The shape of things to come, if you let them. The future is not predictable, but it is shaped by what you do now

David M Conning and Barry D Ricketts

Three trends will influence food purchasing for the next few decades. The first and most dominant of these is convenience. Whether we like it or not, western society – and increasingly other societies that are becoming more urbanized – have become accustomed to enjoying food without the drudgery of meal-preparation, three times daily, day in day out forever. As society becomes more prosperous there will be an upsurge in the provision of ready-made meals or easily prepared alternatives. There will also be an increase in eating out, particularly in fast-food outlets, and the use of snack foods will continue to expand at a substantial rate.

Although there will also be a partial return to the pleasures of elaborate home-cooking, and the joy of the dinner party as social intercourse, these are unlikely to constitute more than a hobby for an affluent minority. What is more likely is that people will meet over a ready-prepared meal bought by the host.

The second trend will be the greater use of new technologies in food preparation, both in the home and in catering. Increasingly sophisticated deep-freezes and microwave ovens will become universal, together with all the paraphernalia designed to reduce the chores inherent in food preparation and waste disposal. There will be comparable advances in industrial technology which will expand the concept and range of convenience food through developments, for example, in extrusion cooking and in food preservation through packing and irradiation.

As a consequence, there is likely to be continued reduction in the use of additives to protect food against spoilage and those used to preserve the cosmetic characteristics of prepared meals. The use of rapid-freezing techniques and controlled-atmosphere packaging will go some way to preserving the volatile flavours that make cooked foods enjoyable and the colours that make them attractive. It could be that the supreme position of canning as a preservation technique will be eroded by flash cooking and freezing, and we will be able to buy packets of deep-frozen cooked vegetables with no added colours and soups with no added flavours.

There is no prospect, however, that the complete range of additives will prove to be dispensable. As we have seen, emulsifiers and stabilizers will be needed and there is no alternative at present to nitrite to prevent botulism. It is also clear that many consumers will require time to adapt to the different forms and textures of foods as processing techniques move towards the physical, and as chemical manipulation is reduced. Indeed it may be that the acceptance of these changes will be the manifestation of a future generation gap.

The third trend will be the provision of better-quality foods which will involve changes in both aesthetic and nutritional quality. Tremendous opportunities exist for retailers of convenience foods, not only to expand the range of meals provided but, by concentrating on the combinations of correct basic ingredients and adapting original recipes to modern processing techniques, to move nearer to the original concepts of taste, texture and presentation. Although initially the price of such meals is likely to be higher than is currently the case, consumers will be prepared to pay the price for greater enjoyment. As the market expands, price differentials will be eroded.

Hand-in-hand with improvements in aesthetic quality will go improvement in nutritional content. There will be opportunity to create meals that are nutritionally balanced within particular energy requirements. To achieve this, other technological developments will occur. For example, the recent development of calorie-free 'fats' is indicative of a field of study that promises to revolutionize the relationship between food science and nutrition. The application of biotechnology has already provided a 'meat substitute' that has proved to be popular with the consumer and has the advantages of reduced energy content and increased fibre. It may be that future developments will result in similar products to limit the energy content of sugars and starches. There is already substantial usage of intense sweeteners in limited applications, but future products are likely to be more versatile. It is possible that with these developments, supplementation of the diet with, for example, vitamins and minerals, will be required. Even fast foods will taste better and be better for you as caterers take advantage of these developments. Many of these changes will be underpinned by progress in plant and animal breeding techniques, directed towards the specific nutritional or aesthetic objectives. These advances are not without attendant risks.

A combination of the power and sophistication of the retailer, and the increasing effectiveness of the consumer movement, has ensured that manufacturers are able to respond rapidly to changes in consumers' perceptions of their needs. This flexibility is more likely to improve than to deteriorate over time, enabling new eating fashions and dietary ingredients to become widely distributed very quickly. This presents problems for two reasons.

First, changing consumer preferences are seldom related to scientific fact. More often, changes are ill-informed, media-driven responses to unproved hypotheses, or worse, cycles of fashionable tastes, dressed up as 'healthy eating' and having little relevance to individual dietary needs. If a dietary trend is of no real benefit to consumers, or worse, has long-term ill-effects, the producer and manufacturer will eventually be blamed, with little regard to the fact that industry was merely responding to the consumers' perception of 'need'. The 'It seemed a good idea at the time' defence is of little avail against 'Industry profiteers while consumers suffer' accusations. Product liability claims will most likely cost manufacturers millions while the main culprit, the media, escape scot-free with two good stories: the introduction of the new wonder-diet, and the subsequent discovery that it is lethal! This may sound far-fetched, but it is merely an extension of what has happened already in certain areas of the diet industry.

Secondly, to change the methods of production and manufacture in order to generate new or different products takes a great deal of ingenuity and investment. Where the change is related to health, manufacturers come under enormous pressure, both moral and political, to act quickly. If the scientific data on which the health claim is based are of dubious quality, there is a natural reluctance to commit large resources to a project that might be found to be based on false assumptions. The industry then comes under further attack for its intransigence.

If manufacturers and those responsible for regulating their activities often appear overly cautious and conservative, it is because the above factors conspire to produce a quite reasonable conviction that they will be wrong, whatever they do! So how can this obstacle to genuine dietary progress be overcome?

Clearly, consumers and those who inform them must stop treating dietary and nutritional matters as subjects of neurotic entertainment – a kind of twentieth-century alchemy – and start learning and respecting a few facts about one of the most vital life sciences of all.

The overweight journalist drowning a stressful morning with a mind-numbing cocktail is hardly the channel through which objective nutritional information is likely to pass to the public. If that stereotype displeases you, what about the teacher who encourages children to reject meat by introducing animal-rights propaganda into the classroom?

The challenge facing educators and communicators is at once formidable and simple. Cease being a conduit for hype, hypotheses, hysteria and plain old-fashioned self-interest. Acquire the information to enable sensible checking of sources; avoid the temptation to pass on propaganda in favour of the challenge to inform and educate.

The public – of whatever age or social status – must learn that good nutrition is a fundamental piece of self-knowledge. It cannot be achieved by slavish adherence to the latest 'healthy eating' fad. The facts are free. The British Nutrition Foundation and a host of other independent sources will willingly help.

It is likely that for the majority, however, the new horizons will represent great opportunities to enhance their perceptions of food quality. Coupled with a better understanding of nutritional matters, eating will be re-established as a central part of human culture in the twenty-first century.

However, if we are to realize the best of our opportunities, the science of nutrition will have to advance a good deal more rapidly than has been apparent in recent years. There are many questions that remain unanswered.

We do not know how to determine if an individual is adequately nourished. Height and weight may be right, but what about calcium levels?

We do not know enough about food choice. Do people eat certain foods because they need certain nutrients, or do they eat any food because they are empty?

If people eat calorie-free foods will they over-compensate? If so, what price dieting?

We do not know enough about different nutrients on body function. Are vitamins tranquillizers?

Does fibre make us euphoric? Is it true that nutrients can be poisonous in the long term?

If we are worried about additives, what about proteins and amino acids?

If sodium chloride is bad, what about magnesium chloride?

Finally, if we get worried about what we know, what about what we don't know?

Such questions may seem contrived, but our diet is governed to a considerable extent by our legislative and regulatory system. New foods or new concepts of eating will have to be assessed by expert committees. How will the experts learn their expertise?

Nutrition science has always been a Cinderella among the biological sciences, and the position is unlikely to improve unless a concerted effort is made at all levels of our education system. Unless nutrition education is started at an early age it is unlikely that enough interest will be generated to last into adulthood. The future lies with our children and it is with them that the preparations should begin.

The search for and appreciation of good nutrition is not the exclusive preserve of any group, clique, industry or ministry. If we are to attain the many rich benefits to be achieved from being well-nourished, whether young or old, affluent or deprived, then we must *all* share in the investment.

Appendices

Glossary of Diet and Nutrition

acceptable daily intake (ADI)   the maximum permitted level of a chemical in the diet (one-hundredth of the no-effect level)

acetic acid   the main component of vinegar; used as a preservative

acid   substance which neutralizes alkali; strong solutions may be caustic or corrosive

adipose   fatty

adipose tissue   tissue storing fat

aesthetics   perceived qualities; includes texture, flavour, presentation, etc., of food

agar   polysaccharide extracted from red seaweed; used as a thickener and stabilizer

albumin   protein; one of the major dissolved components in blood and also plentiful in egg white; used as an emulsifier and stabilizer

alkali (base)   substance which neutralizes acid; strong solutions may be caustic or corrosive

allergen   substance which provokes an allergic reaction in a sensitive individual, e.g. certain foods, grass pollen, etc.

allergy   exaggerated reaction of the immune system to an otherwise harmless substance; symptoms range from a rash to breathing difficulties

amino acid   molecules containing nitrogen, a carboxyl (acidic) group and a side chain attached to a single carbon atom; about twenty are found in nature; used to build proteins

amino group   molecule consisting of a nitrogen atom with hydrogen atoms joined to it

amylase enzyme produced in saliva and pancreatic juices which breaks down starch into smaller units for further digestion

anabolic agents substances which tend to promote tissue growth by increasing protein synthesis

anabolic steroid hormone used as an anabolic agent; usually a male sex hormone

anaemia condition where the levels of haemoglobin, the main oxygen-carrying component of the blood, are low; may be caused by low dietary intake of iron, vitamin B_{12} or folic acid

angina pectoris pain in the chest caused by a lack of oxygen supply to the heart, usually brought on by exertion or excitement

anorexia loss of or poor appetite

anorexia nervosa eating disorder with a psychological component associated with severe restriction of food intake and emaciation

antibody specialized protein formed in the body by the immune system to combine with, and to render harmless, a particular foreign substance known as an antigen

antigen foreign protein or protein-polysaccharide which will bring about an immune response, e.g. the formation of antibodies

antimicrobial substance that injures or kills microorganisms such as bacteria, fungi or viruses

antioxidant substance which combines with oxygen to prevent potentially harmful effects; used to stop rancidity in fats

ascorbic acid (vitamin C) substance found in citrus fruits, salad vegetables, potatoes and liver and needed by the body for healthy supporting tissues; used as an antioxidant

aseptic free from microorganisms; achieved by sterilization

aspartame artificial sweetener with little or no energy content, derived from two amino acids; 180 times sweeter than sucrose

atheroma deposit formed of muscle cells, cholesterol and connective tissue on the inner wall of an artery

atherosclerosis disease characterized by atheroma, leading to narrowing of the arteries and potentially to obstruction of blood-flow

atom smallest particle of elements which can take part in a chemical change; made up of protons (positively charged), electrons (negatively charged) and neutrons (neutrally charged)

bacteria *see* microorganisms

basal metabolic rate (BMR) measurement of the energy required to perform those basic functions needed to maintain life, e.g. breathing, liver function

benzoic acid organic acid used as a preservative

blanch immerse briefly in hot water or steam to inactivate enzymes which cause deterioration; prepare for canning or freezing

BMR *see* basal metabolic rate

botulism serious form of food poisoning caused by the *Clostridium botulinum* bacteria which produce a toxin

bran outer husk of grain which provides a rich source of dietary fibre and also contains phytic acid

bulimia eating disorder with a psychological component associated with the consumption of huge amounts of food, followed by self-induced vomiting and/or purging

calcium mineral found particularly in dairy products and needed for the building and maintenance of strong bones and teeth; absorption is dependent on vitamin D

calcium carbonate (chalk) substance added to white flour to increase level of calcium

calipers instrument for the measurement of skinfold thickness which is used to estimate total body fat

calorie amount of heat required to raise the temperature of one gram of water by one degree Celsius; used to measure the energy contained in food. We often use the term 'calorie' when really we mean one kilocalorie or one Calorie (1000 calories). *See also* joule.

cancer uncontrolled growth or malformation of cells which can lead to illness and, possibly, death

CAP *see* Common Agriculture Policy

caramelization heating of sugar to a temperature above its melting point, giving rise to a range of golden-brown products

carbohydrate class of molecules made of carbon, hydrogen and oxygen with the hydrogen and oxygen atoms in the same proportions as in water; may be subdivided into mono-, di- and polysaccharides. Most are digested by the body to provide energy.

carboxyl group molecule consisting of a carbon atom bonded to two oxygen atoms and either a hydrogen atom or some side chain; the essential chemical group of organic acids

carcinogenic leading to or associated with cancer

carotene member of the carotenoid family; precursor of vitamin A

carotenoids group of pigments which produce the yellow and orange colours of some fruits and vegetables

carrageenan polysaccharide extracted from seaweed and used in gel form as an emulsifier and stabilizer

cellulose polysaccharide of plant origin which is not digested in the human gut; used as an emulsifier and stabilizer and can form membranes such as sausage skins

centrifuge spin a mixture, separating it into components of different density

cerebrovascular disease disease affecting blood vessels in the brain, e.g. stroke

chemical relating to chemistry; also used to describe molecules, e.g. salt is a chemical called sodium chloride

chemistry science of the elements and their laws of combination

chlorine dioxide gas used as a bleaching agent in flour

cholesterol lipid substance manufactured in the body and found in most foods of animal origin; required for synthesis of cell membranes

Clostridium botulinum bacterium which grows in badly-preserved canned foods, producing a toxin which causes serious food-poisoning

collagen protein which provides structural support in tissues, e.g. tendons in humans

Common Agricultural Policy (CAP) policy of the EEC designed to ensure adequate food supplies and adequate payment to farmers

coronary (ischaemic heart disease) group of conditions associated with low oxygen supply to the heart tissue; include angina pectoris, myocardial infarction and sudden death

curd clotted protein formed when rennet is added to fresh milk; when sweetened and flavoured it is known as junket

dehydrate remove water; preserve food by making it hard for microorganisms to survive

denature disorganize irreversibly the arrangement of protein chains, usually by heating

dental caries tooth decay due to the action of acid formed from carbohydrate digestion by bacteria in the mouth

dental plaque soft non-mineralized bacterial deposit on teeth which forms if they are not adequately cleaned

DES *see* diethylstilboestrol

dextrin carbohydrate formed as an intermediary product during the digestion of starch

diabetes mellitus (sugar diabetes) disease associated with an inability to maintain blood glucose levels within the normal range, due to a lack of insulin or resistance to its actions

dietary fibre group of substances not broken down by the digestive enzymes in humans; main constituents are cellulose, lignin, pectin and gums

diethylstilboestrol (DES) synthetic female hormone used to fatten livestock; now banned because it may cause cancer

digestion process of breaking down foodstuffs into simpler components that can be absorbed and used by the body

diglyceride   lipid molecule wherein fatty acids are attached to two of the three carbon atoms of glycerol

disaccharide   carbohydrate molecule made up of two monosaccharides, e.g. sucrose is made of glucose and fructose

emulsifier   substance, usually a long molecule with one end lipid-soluble and the other end water-soluble, which facilitates the formation of an emulsion

emulsion   fine mixture of two liquids which normally would not mix, such as oil and water

endosperm   inner part of any grain; a store of starch

energy   the ability to perform work; can neither be created nor destroyed, but can be changed from one form to another. The energy of foods is expressed in kilocalories or kilojoules (*see* calorie, joule)

energy balance   term used to describe the matching of energy consumption and energy expenditure

enzyme   protein which increases the rate of (catalyses) a specific biochemical reaction without itself being used up; many thousands of enzymes are found in the body, each doing a particular job. Many enzymes work together to produce 'chain' reactions

essential fatty acid   fatty acid which must be obtained from the diet because it cannot be synthesized in the human body

esters   products of the combination of alcohols with organic acids; fats are esters of fatty acids and glycerol

ethylene gas (ethene)   organic gas which stimulates ripening of fruit and is used to fumigate grain

extrusion   formation of a food product by forcing a paste, usually of starch, through perforated steel plates, e.g. pasta, cereal products

extrusion cooking   cooking of a food product as it is extruded

fat   class of lipid molecules made of a glycerol backbone with up to three fatty acids attached; usually solids, whereas oils are usually liquids

fatty acid   chain of carbon atoms with a carboxyl group at one end; over 40 are found in nature; subdivided according to the number of double bonds between carbon atoms, i.e. none if unsaturated, one if monounsaturated and more than one if polyunsaturated

foam   mixture of a gas, usually air, within a liquid

folic acid   vitamin of the B complex found in dark-green vegetables, oranges, avocado pears, wholegrain cereals, liver and kidney; required in the synthesis of DNA, the genetic material of cells

freeze-drying   technique of freezing and drying food which combines the advantages of both processes, resulting in a light and compact product that can be stored at room temperature

fructose (fruit sugar)   simple sugar molecule which is found free in only a few foods, such as honey, apples and pears; nearly twice as sweet as sucrose

fuller's earth   porous earth which readily absorbs grease and can be used in the refining of oils and fats

galactose   simple sugar molecule which is found combined with glucose as lactose or milk sugar

gelatinize   form a gel; heat starch in water so that its granules swell up and eventually burst, producing a gel which may be used as a thickener

germ (embryo)   is the shoot and root of a grain; contains oil, protein, vitamins and minerals

glucose   simple sugar molecule found free in fruits and vegetables or combined in sucrose and starch; about half as sweet as sucrose; the principal sugar in animals

gluten   protein found in wheat, rye and in smaller amounts in barley and oats; has elastic properties and traps gas when it expands; essential in bread- and cake-making

glyceride   general term for fat referring to glycerol molecules with one or more fatty acids attached

glycerol   molecule made in the body which forms part of the structure of fats; may be used as a solvent

gum polysaccharide usually found in plants; though not itself fibrous, it forms part of dietary fibre, used as thickener, stabilizer and emulsifier. There are many different kinds of gums, depending on origin, chemical structure, etc.

heart attack what occurs when a diseased coronary artery becomes blocked and the heart muscle is suddenly deprived of blood; characterized by sudden chest pain, breathlessness, etc., may be immediately fatal

hormonal replacement therapy (HRT) use of very small doses of female hormones to alleviate the effects of the menopause

hormone 'messenger' molecules produced in glands which travel in the blood to stimulate actions in other parts of the body

HRT *see* hormonal replacement therapy

hydrogen inflammable gas; the lightest element; present in all things that live or have lived

hydrogenation process of adding hydrogen atoms to molecules; artificial saturation of oils used in the production of margarine

hydrolysis reaction in which molecules are changed by the chemical addition of water

hyperactivity rare condition of extreme restlessness and inattentiveness in children, which can result in disruptive behaviour and underachievement

hyperglycaemia high blood-glucose level which may be associated with excessive hunger, thirst and urination; the basic problem in untreated diabetes mellitus (due to lack of insulin or resistance to its actions)

hypertension (high blood-pressure) condition common in middle-aged and elderly people; recognized as a risk factor for coronary heart disease

hypoglycaemia low blood-glucose level which may be associated with hunger, sweating and headaches; if severe and untreated can lead to coma or death; one of the problems that may arise in the treatment of diabetes mellitus

ideal body-weight   desirable range of weight for an individual according to his/her height. A body-weight within this range is associated with the best chance of a long life

immune system   group of cells and cell products (such as antibodies) used by the body to cope with foreign substances; major defence against bacteria and viruses

inositol   chemical present in many foods, especially bran and cereals; member of the alcohol group of chemicals

insulin   protein hormone produced in the pancreas, which controls the uptake and release of glucose; also important in protein and fat metabolism

inversion   conversion of sucrose into glucose and fructose, producing a mixture which is not crystalline. Honey is very largely 'inverted' sucrose. The name derives from the change in the way light is deflected.

ion   charged particle formed when an atom loses or gains electrons

irradiation   preservation of food by passing it over a radioactive source; used to prevent bacterial infection and to delay ripening

joule   unit of measurement applicable to all forms of energy, including work and heat; one calorie equals 4.2 joules

kilocalorie (Calorie)   unit of energy measurement equal to 1000 calories

lactic acid   organic acid produced in the anaerobic metabolism of glucose; such conditions of low oxygen are found in industrial fermentation or within the body during exercise; used as a preservative

lactose or milk sugar   disaccharide composed of glucose and galactose

lacto-ovo-vegetarian   vegetarian who eats dairy products and eggs

lacto-vegetarian   vegetarian who eats dairy products such as milk and cheese, but not eggs

lecithin   lipid molecule made in the body and found in vegetable oils, seeds and egg yolk; used as an emulsifier

linoleic acid   essential, polyunsaturated fatty acid

lipid   biochemical term for fatty substances, e.g. fat, cholesterol and lecithin

lipoprotein   protein with a lipid incorporated into its structure, found in the blood, cell membranes, etc.; very important in all biological tissues and processes

lumen   inner open space or bore in a tube or other walled cavity

maltose   disaccharide composed of two glucose molecules; formed by the breakdown of starch and present in small amounts in malted foods

mannitol   sugar alcohol used as an artificial sweetener

metabolism   general term for chemical processes which occur in the body, including the building up of complex molecules from simple ones and the breaking down of complex molecules into simple ones, with the release of energy

microorganism   very small living creature invisible to the naked eye, such as bacteria and viruses

molecule   two or more atoms joined chemically or bonded together

monoglyceride   lipid molecule wherein a fatty acid is attached to one of the carbon atoms of glycerol

monosaccharide   carbohydrate molecule; the simplest form of sugar, e.g. glucose, galactose and fructose

monosodium glutamate (MSG)   an amino acid found in most living cells and used as a flavour-enhancer for food

MSG   *see* monosodium glutamate

myocardial infarction   death of part of the heart tissue due to insufficient oxygen, produced by a failure of blood supply; may be associated with severe chest pain and can be fatal

niacin   vitamin of the B complex found in meat, fortified breakfast cereals, fruits and vegetables; used in the liberation of energy within cells

nitrates and nitrites preservatives particularly effective against *Clostridium botulinum*

no-effect level highest dose of a chemical which produces *no* effect in the animal to which it is fed over the lifetime of that animal

non-dairy creamer product based on filled milk used to whiten tea and coffee

non-essential amino or fatty acid an amino or fatty acid that can be synthesized by the body and therefore need not be taken in the diet

nutrient food substance providing energy and the raw material for the synthesis and maintenance of cells in the body, comprising fat, carbohydrate, protein, vitamins and minerals; water and oxygen are essential to life but are not nutrients

obesity condition in which a person's weight is more than 20% greater than the ideal body-weight predicted from his/her height, the excess being due to fat, rather than muscle or bone

organic acid acid present in or derived from living tissues; containing a carboxyl group

osteoporosis condition of reduced bone density which may cause bones to break more easily; associated with calcium loss and decreased production of ovarian hormones after menopause

overweight condition in which a person's weight is more than 10% greater than the ideal body-weight predicted from his/her height

oxidation process involving addition of oxygen or removal of hydrogen

parboil steam for a few minutes to inactivate enzymes and to soften; when rice is parboiled, thiamin is driven into the grain so that it is not all lost when the cereal is milled

pasteurization process of heating, then cooling, raw milk in order to kill some of the bacteria which cause disease and spoilage

pathogen disease-causing organisms, e.g. bacteria

pectin polysaccharide found in plants which forms part of dietary fibre, though it is not itself fibrous; can form gels; used as a stabilizer

phenol   organic substance that can be used as an antiseptic

phospholipid   lipid molecule formed from glycerol esterified to two fatty acids and a phosphate molecule; the main structural lipid in cell membranes

phytic acid   molecule composed of inositol and phosphorus, found in nuts, wholegrain cereals and pulses; will form insoluble salts with calcium, iron and zinc, thereby interfering with their absorption

polyphosphates   substances used as additives to prevent the normal loss of water from meats on cooking

polysaccharide   large carbohydrate molecule built up from monosaccharides joined in long chains which may be straight or branched, e.g. starch or cellulose

polyunsaturated fatty acid (PUFA)   fatty acid containing two or more double bonds between its carbon atoms; examples include the essential fatty acids

potassium bromate   food additive used in bread-making

preservative   substance added to food to slow down the process of deterioration, e.g. by preventing bacterial contamination

protein   class of large molecules which are made from chains of amino acids; form the basis of structural tissues as well as acting as regulators of function (as hormones and enzymes) and may also be used as an energy source

PUFA   *see* polyunsaturated fatty acid

RDA   *see* recommended daily allowance

recommended daily allowance (RDA)   lists issued by governments and WHO of amounts of various nutrients which are likely to meet the needs of most people in the population

rennet   commercial preparation of the enzyme rennin which is extracted from calves' stomachs or from vegetable sources; used in the clotting of milk and making of cheese and curds

rickets   disease associated with deformity of the bones caused by insufficient absorption of calcium, due to a lack of vitamin D

saccharin   artificial non-calorific sweetener up to 500 times as sweet as sucrose

salmonella   group of bacteria whose members are mainly found in the intestinal tract of animals and humans; cause illness including food poisoning and typhoid fever; will multiply in foods which have been inadequately cooked; infection can be transferred to cooked foods from a contaminated raw-food source via kitchen staff or utensils

saltpetre (sodium nitrate)   preservative used in pickling meat, which produces a pink colour

saturated fatty acid   fatty acid with no double bonds between its carbon atoms, i.e. contains a full complement of hydrogen atoms

scurvy   disease caused by severe dietary deficiency of vitamin C in which the body's supporting tissues become weakened

serum   blood plasma which has clotted and from which the clot has been removed

sodium bicarbonate   compound which reacts with acid to produce carbon dioxide gas; *see* tartaric acid

sodium carbonate   substance used to control acidity in jam

sodium chloride   common salt; one of the earliest preservatives

sorbitol   sugar alcohol used as an artificial sweetener

spores   dormant form of microorganisms (e.g. bacteria) which are able to withstand lack of water and extremes of temperature until conditions are suitable for growth and reproduction

stabilizer   substance used to maintain an emulsion, suspension or foam in the desired state

starch   polysaccharide formed from long chains of glucose molecules; storage form of glucose in plants and an important source of energy in the diet

sterilization   means of rendering objects, wounds, etc. free from microorganisms which can cause disease or spoilage; a rigorous heat treatment of milk which improves keeping quality but affects flavour adversely

stroke   consequence of an interruption of blood-supply to the brain, often caused by a blood clot; may result in paralysis

sucrose   carbohydrate molecule made up of fructose and glucose

sulphites   substances derived from sulphur and used as antimicrobials in wine-making and fruit- or vegetable-preserving

sulphur dioxide   gas used as a preservative

suspension   mixture of solid and liquid wherein particles of the former are dispersed in the latter

synthesis   formation of compounds by chemistry

tartaric acid   substance used as potassium tartrate to release carbon dioxide from sodium bicarbonate in baking powders and self-raising flour

thiamin (vitamin B$_1$)   vitamin found in wholegrain cereals, nuts, beans, milk and yeast extract; used in the release of energy from carbohydrates

toxin   poisonous substance

triglyceride   molecule wherein fatty acids are attached to all three carbon atoms of glycerol; a 'simple fat'

trypsin inhibitor   substance found in raw soya beans which limits the ability of the enzyme trypsin to digest proteins

UHT   *see* ultra-high-temperature

ultra-high-temperature (UHT)   treatment for milk which heats it to high temperatures for a short time, allowing it a shelf-life of up to six months

underweight   condition in which a person's weight is below the ideal body-weight predicted from his/her height

unsaturated fatty acid   fatty acid containing one or more double bonds between its carbon atoms

vegan   vegetarian who does not eat any produce of animal origin

vegetarian   person who does not eat the flesh of animals, i.e. meat or fish, and may also exclude dairy products and/or eggs from his/her diet

virus extremely small microorganism which cannot replicate without using a host cell; sometimes causes disease

vitamin a type of nutrient; diverse group of organic substances needed for growth and metabolism. They cannot be synthesized by the body in sufficient amounts and must therefore be supplied by the diet

whey fluid that separates from clot in cheese-making; contains most of the lactose and almost no casein, protein or fat

'E' Numbers Identified

To find a particular additive on this list, look first at its category as listed on the label – for example, Colour or Preservative. Additives are listed in numerical order *within* each category. Those without numbers are listed alphabetically at the end of each section. The list also tries to give an idea of foods in which each additive is used. Many additives can be used for similar functions. These additives are listed together in tinted boxes. Examples of foods in which they might be used are given at the bottom of each box. The uses given are merely examples – they do not represent the only uses to which the additives are put nor are they meant to imply that these are the only uses allowed by law.

Antioxidants
Stop fatty foods from going rancid and protect fat-soluble vitamins from the harmful effects of oxidation.

E300	**L-ascorbic acid** fruit drinks; also used to improve flour and bread dough
E301	**sodium L-ascorbate**
E302	**calcium L-ascorbate**
E304	**6-0-palmitoyl-L-ascorbic acid (ascorbyl palmitate)** scotch eggs
E306	**extracts of natural origin rich in tocopherols** vegetable oils
E307	**synthetic alpha-tocopherol** cereal-based baby foods
E308	**synthetic gamma-tocopherol**
E309	**synthetic delta-tocopherol**
E310	**propyl gallate** vegetable oils; chewing gum
E311	**octyl gallate**
E312	**dodecyl gallate**
E320	**butylated hydroxyanisole (BHA)** beef stock cubes; cheese spread

E321   **butylated hydroxytoluene (BHT)** chewing gum

E322   **lecithins** low fat spreads; also used as an emulsifier in chocolate
         diphenylamine
         ethoxyquin used to prevent 'scald' (a discolouration) on apples and pears

Colours

Make food more colourful, compensate for colour lost in processing.

E100   **curcumin** flour confectionery, margarine

E101   **riboflavin** sauces

101(a) **riboflavin-5′-phosphate**

E102   **tartrazine** soft drinks

E104   **quinoline yellow**

107   **yellow 2G**

E110   **sunset yellow FCF** biscuits

E120   **cochineal** alcoholic drinks

E122   **carmoisine** jams and preserves

E123   **amaranth**

E124   **ponceau 4R** dessert mixes

E127   **erythrosine** glacé cherries

128   **red 2G** sausages

E131   **patent blue V**

E132   **indigo carmine**

133   **brilliant blue FCF** canned vegetables

E140   **chlorophyll**

E141   **copper complexes of chlorophyll and chlorophyllins**

E142   **green S** pastilles

E150   **caramel** beer, soft drinks, sauces, gravy browning

E151   **black PN**

E153   **carbon black (vegetable carbon)** liquorice

154   **brown FK** kippers

155   **brown HT (chocolate brown HT)** chocolate cake

160(a) **alpha-carotene; beta-carotene; gamma-carotene** margarine, soft drinks

E160(b) **annatto; bixin; norbixin** crisps

E160(a) **capsanthin; capsorubin**

E160(d) **lycopene**

E160(e) **beta-apo-8′-carotenal**

E160(f) **ethyl ester of beta-apo-8′-carotenoic acid**

E161(a) **flavoxanthin**

E161(b) lutein
E161(c) cryptoxanthin
E161(d) rubixanthin
E161(e) violaxanthin
E161(f) rhodoxanthin
E161(g) canthaxanthin
E162   beetroot red (betanin)   ice-cream, liquorice
E163   anthocyanins   yoghurt
E171   titanium dioxide   sweets
E172   iron oxides; iron hydroxides
E173   aluminium
E174   silver
E175   gold   cake decorations
E180   pigment rubine (lithol rubine BK)

methyl violet   used for the surface marking of citrus fruit

paprika   canned vegetables

saffron; crocin

sandalwood; santolin

turmeric   soups

Emulsifiers and stabilizers

Enable oils and fats to mix with water in foods; add to smoothness and creaminess of texture; retard baked goods going stale.

E400   alginic acid   ice-cream; soft cheese
E401   sodium alginate   cake mixes
E402   potassium alginate
E403   ammonium alginate
E404   calcium alginate
E405   propane-1,2-diol alginate (propylene glycol alginate)   salad dressings; cottage cheese
E406   agar   ice-cream
E407   carrageenan   quick setting jelly mixes; milk shakes
E410   locust bean gum (carob gum)   salad cream
E412   guar gum   packet soups and meringue mixes
E413   tragacanth   salad dressings; processed cheese
E414   gum arabic (acacia)   confectionery
E415   xanthan gum   sweet pickle; coleslaw
416   karaya gum   soft cheese; brown sauce
430   polyoxyethylene (8) stearate

431   polyoxyethylene (40) stearate

432   polyoxyethylene (20) sorbitan monolaurate (Polysorbate 20)

433   polyoxyethylene (20) sorbitan mono-oleate (Polysorbate 80)

434   polyoxyethylene (20) sorbitan monopalmitate (Polysorbate 40)

435   polyoxyethylene (20) sorbitan monostearate (Polysorbate 60)

436   polyoxyethylene (20) sorbitan tristearate (Polysorbate 65)   bakery products; confectionery creams

E440(a) pectin

E440(b) amidated pectin
        pectin extract   jams and preserves

442   **ammonium phosphatides** cocoa and chocolate products

E460   **microcrystalline cellulose; alpha-cellulose (powdered cellulose)** high-fibre bread; grated cheese

E461   **methylcellulose** low fat spreads

E463   **hydroxypropylcellulose**

E464   **hydroxypropylmethylcellulose** edible ices

E465   **ethylmethylcellulose** gateaux

E466   **carboxymethylcellulose, sodium salt (CMC)** jelly, gateaux

E470   **sodium, potassium and calcium salts of fatty acids** cake mixes

E471   **mono- and di-glycerides of fatty acids** frozen desserts

E472(a) **acetic esters of mono- and di-glycerides of fatty acids** mousse mixes

E472(b) **lactic acid esters of mono- and di-glycerides of fatty acids** dessert topping

E472(c) **citric acid esters of mono- and di-glycerides of fatty acids** continental sausages

E472(e) **mono- and diacetyltartaric acid esters of mono- and di-glycerides of fatty acids** bread; frozen pizza

E473   **sucrose esters of fatty acids**

E474   **sucroglycerides** edible ices

E475   **polyglycerol esters of fatty acids** cakes and gateaux

476   **polyglycerol esters of polycondensed fatty acids of castor oil (polyglycerol polyricinoleate)** chocolate-flavour coatings for cakes

E477   propane-1,2-diol esters of fatty acids instant desserts

478   lactylated fatty acid esters of glycerol and propane-1,2-diol

E481   sodium stearoyl-2-lactylate bread, cakes and biscuits

E482   calcium stearoyl-2-lactylate gravy granules

E483   stearyl tartrate

491   sorbitan monostearate

492   sorbitan tristearate

493   sorbitan monolaurate

494   sorbitan mono-oleate

495   sorbitan monopalmitate cake mixes

dioctyl sodium sulphosuccinate used in sugar refining to help crystallization

extracts of quillaia used in soft drinks to promote foam

oxidatively polymerised soya bean oil

polyglycerol esters of dimerised fatty acids of soya bean oil emulsions used to grease bakery tins

Preservatives

Protect food against microbes which cause spoilage and food poisoning. They also increase storage life of foods.

E200   sorbic acid soft drinks; fruit yoghurt; processed cheese slices

E201   sodium sorbate

E202   potassium sorbate

E203   calcium sorbate frozen pizza; flour confectionery

E210   benzoic acid

E211   sodium benzoate

E212   potassium benzoate

E213   calcium benzoate

E214   ethyl 4-hydroxybenzoate (ethyl para-hydroxy-benzoate)

E215   ethyl 4-hydroxybenzoate, sodium salt (sodium ethyl para-hydroxybenzoate)

E216   propyl 4-hydroxybenzoate (propyl para-hydroxy-benzoate)

E217   propyl 4-hydroxybenzoate, sodium salt (sodium propyl para-hydroxybenzoate)

E218   methyl 4-hydroxybenzoate (methyl para-hydroxybenzoate)

E219   methyl 4-hydroxybenzoate, sodium salt (sodium methyl para-hydroxybenzoate) beer, jam, salad cream, soft drinks, fruit pulp, fruit-based pie fillings, marinated herring and mackerel

E220   sulphur dioxide

E221   sodium sulphite

E222   sodium hydrogen sulphite (sodium bisulphite)

E223   sodium metabisulphite

E224   potassium metabisulphite

E226   calcium sulphite

E227   calcium hydrogen sulphite (calcium bisulphite) dried fruit, dehydrated vegetables, fruit juices and syrups, sausages, fruit-based dairy desserts, cider, beer and wine; also used to prevent browning of raw peeled potatoes and to condition biscuit doughs

E230   biphenyl(diphenyl)

E231   2-hydroxybiphenyl(orthophenylphenol)

E232   sodium biphenyl-2-yl oxide (sodium orthophenyl-phenate) surface treatment of citrus fruit

E233   2-(thiazol-4-yl) benzimidazole (thiabendazole) surface treatment of bananas

234   nisin   cheese, clotted cream

E239   hexamine   (hexamethylenetetramine) marinated herring and mackerel

E249   potassium nitrite

E250   sodium nitrite

E251   sodium nitrate

E252   potassium nitrate   bacon, ham, cured meats, corned beef and some cheeses

E280   propionic acid

E281   sodium propionate

E282   calcium propionate

E283   potassium propionate bread and flour confectionery, Christmas pudding

Sweeteners

There are two types of sweeteners – intense sweeteners and bulk sweeteners. Intense sweeteners have a sweetness many times that of sugar and are therefore used at very low levels: They are marked with '*' in the list below. Bulk sweeteners have about the same sweetness as sugar and are used at the same sort of levels as sugar.

	* acesulfame potassium	canned foods, soft drinks, table-top sweeteners
	* aspartame	soft drinks, yoghurts, dessert and drink mixes, sweetening tablets
	hydrogenated glucose syrup	
	isomalt	
E421	**mannitol**	sugar-free confectionery
	* saccharin	
	* sodium saccharin	
	* calcium saccharin	soft drinks, cider, sweetening tablets, table-top sweeteners
E420	**sorbitol; sorbitol syrup**	sugar-free confectionery, jams for diabetics
	* thaumatin	table-top sweeteners, yoghurt
	xylitol	sugar-free chewing gum

Taken from FOOD ADDITIVES: THE BALANCED APPROACH.
Reproduced with the permission of the Controller of Her Majesty's Stationery Office.

Useful Addresses

Advertising Standards Authority
Brook House
2–16 Torrington Place
London WC1E 7HN
Tel: 01 580 5555

Allinsons
Healthways House
45 Station Approach
West Byfleet
Surrey KT14 6NE
Tel: 0932 341133

Association of Agriculture
Victoria Chambers 16/20 Strutton Ground
London SW1P 2HP
Tel: 01 222 6115/6

British Diabetic Association
10 Queen Anne Street
London W1M 0BD
Tel: 01 323 1531

British Farm Produce Council
417/418 Market Towers
New Covent Garden Market
London SW8 5NQ

British Heart Foundation
102 Gloucester Place
London W1H 4DH
Tel: 01 935 0185

British Independent Grocers Association
Federation House
17 Farnborough Street
Hants GU14 8AG
Tel: 0252 515001

British Meat
Educational Service
5 St John's Square
London EC1M 4DE
Tel. 01 251 2021

British Nutrition Foundation
15 Belgrave Square
London SW1X 8PS
Tel: 01 235 4904

Butter Information Council Ltd
Tubs Hill House
London Road
Sevenoaks
Kent TN13 1BL
Tel: 0732 460060

The Coeliac Society
P O Box 220
High Wycombe
Bucks HP11 2HY

Consumers Association
14 Buckingham Street
London WC2N 6DS
Tel: 01 839 1222

Coronary Prevention Group
60 Great Ormond Street
London WC1N 3HR
Tel: 01 833 3687

Dairy Produce Advisory Service
Milk Marketing Board
Thames Ditton
Surrey KT7 0EL
Tel: 01 398 4101

Department of the Environment
2 Marsham Street
London SW1P 3EB

Department of Health and Social Security
Alexander Fleming House
Elephant & Castle
London SE1 6B9

Department of Trade and Industry
1 Victoria Street
London SW1H 0HT

Farm and Food Society
4 Willifield Way
London NW11
Tel: 01 455 0634

Federation of Wholesale Distributors
18 Fleet Street
London EC4Y 1AS
Tel: 01 353 8894

Flora Project for Heart Disease Prevention
24–28 Bloomsbury Way
London WC1A 2PX
Tel: 01 242 0936

Flour Advisory Bureau
21 Arlington Street
London SW1A 1RN
Tel: 01 493 2521

Food and Drink Federation
6 Catherine Street
London WC2B 5JJ
Tel: 01 836 2460

Fresh Fruit and Vegetable Information Bureau
126–8 Cromwell Road
London SW7 4ET
Tel: 01 373 7734

Friends of the Earth
26 Underwood Street
London N1
Tel: 01 490 1555

Good Housekeeping Institute
National Magazine House
72 Broadwick Street
London W1V 2BP
Tel: 01 439 7144

Home and Freezer Digest
Glenthorne House
Hammersmith Grove
London W6 0LG
Tel: 01 846 9922

John West Foods Ltd
Education Service
10 Barb Mews
London W6 7PA
Tel: 01 602 0958

Kelloggs
Consumer Service Department
Park Road
Stretford
Manchester M32 8RA
Tel: 061 865 4411

London Food Commission
88 Old Street
London EC1V 9AR
Tel: 01 253 9513

Microwave Association
2 Lansdowne House
Lansdowne Road
London W11 3LP
Tel: 01 229 8225

Ministry of Agriculture, Fisheries and Food (MAFF)
Great Westminster House
Horseferry Road
London SW1P 2AE
Tel: 01 216 7444/7343

Mother Earth UK Ltd
80 High Street
London SE25
Tel: 01 771 4391

National Consumer Council
20 Grosvenor Gardens
London SW1W 0DH
Tel: 01 730 3469

National Farmers Union
Agriculture House
Knightsbridge
London SW1X 7NJ
Tel: 01 235 5077

Retail Consortium
Commonwealth House
1–19 New Oxford Street
London WC1A 1PA
Tel: 01 404 4622

Royal College of Physicians
11 St Andrews Place
Regent's Park
London NW1 4LE
Tel: 01 035 1174

Sea Fish Industry Authority
10 Young Street   14 Cromwell Road
Edinburgh EH2 4JQ   London SW7 4ES
Tel: 031 225 2515   Tel: 01373 7273/8495

The Vegetarian Society
Parkdale
Dunham Road
Altrincham
Cheshire WA14 4QG
Tel: 061 928 0793

Bibliography by Topic

The Food Industry
The Food Industry, J Burns, J McInerney, A Swinbank, published in association with the Commonwealth Agricultural Bureau, Heinemann, London, 1983.

A Handbook of Food Packaging, F Paine & H Paine, Leonard Hill, London, 1983.

Food Science
Food Tables, A E Bender & D A Bender, Oxford University Press, Oxford, 1986.

The Composition of Foods, McCance and Widdowson, 4th rev. ed., A A Paul & D A T Southgate, HMSO, London, 1979.

The Science of Food, P M Gamman & K B Sherrington, Pergamon Press, 1977.

Food Additives
The New E For Additives, Maurice Hanssen, Thorsons, Wellingborough, 1987.

Danger! Additives at Work, Melanie Miller, London Food Commission, London, 1985.

Handbook of Food Additives, CRC Press, 1972.

Food and the Consumer
The Food Labelling Debate, Adriana Luba, London Food Commission, London, 1985.

Food Policy and the Consumer, National Consumer Council, London, 1988.

Home Cooking
The Shorter Mrs Beeton, Ward Lock.

French Provincial Cooking, Elizabeth David, Penguin, Harmondsworth.

Classic Italian Cookbook, Marcella Hazan, Macmillan, London.

Classic Indian Cooking, Julie Sahni, Dorling Kindersley, London.

Chinese Food, Kenneth Lo, Penguin, Harmondsworth.

A New Book of Middle Eastern Food, Claudia Roden, Penguin, Harmondsworth.

The Book of Latin American Cookery, Elisabeth Lambert Ortiz, Heinemann, London.

Freezer Facts, Margaret Leach, Forbes Publications Ltd, 1975.

The ABC of Home Freezing, HMSO Bulletin 214, HMSO, London, 1978.

Food Manufacture

Food Processing and Nutrition, A E Bender, Academic Press, 1978.

Food Processing – A Nutritional Perspective, BNF Briefing Paper No. 11, BNF, 1987.

The Science and Technology of Foods, R K Proudlove, Forbes Publications Ltd, 1985.

Food Industries Manual, ed. M D Ranken, Leonard Hill, 1984.

Food in Health and Disease

Eat Your Heart Out, J LeFanu, Macmillan, London, 1987.

Food and Health, Richard Cottrell (ed.), BNF, London, 1987.

Pure, White and Deadly, John Yudkin, Viking, Harmondsworth, 1986.

The Diet of Reason, Digby Anderson, The Social Affairs Unit, 1986.

General

The Manual of Nutrition, Ministry of Agriculture, Fisheries and Food, HMSO, London, 1985.

Eating for Health, Department of Health and Social Security, HMSO, London, 1978.

The English – a social history, Christopher Hibbert, Grafton Books, 1987.

Technological Eating, Magnus Pyke, John Murray, 1972.

On Food and Cooking – the Science and Lore of the Kitchen, Harold McGee, Allen & Unwin, 1984.

Food Intolerance – Fact and Fiction, Dr Juliet Gray, Grafton Books, 1986.

Index

A NEW, MORE SENSIBLE AND HEALTHIER WAY
OF EATING FOR THE ENTIRE FAMILY

MARY BERRY
Feed your family the healthier way!

Mary Berry takes the mystery out of healthy eating
and shows you how to change your family's diet without
them even noticing. She indicates the foods that really
are good for your family, as well as simple, economical
recipes that will have them asking for more.

FEED YOUR FAMILY THE HEALTHIER WAY contains
an easy guide to selecting and preparing more
nutritious foods, helpful hints for introducing natural
foods like brown rice and wholemeal flour into your
family's diet and 175 delicious recipes for everything
from breakfast to puddings. Mary Berry makes good
eating easy.

COOKERY/HEALTH   0 7221 1641 1   £2.95

Also by Mary Berry in Sphere Books:

FAST CAKES	FAST SUPPERS
FRUIT FARE	FAST DESSERTS
FAST STARTERS, SOUPS &	NEW FREEZER COOKBOOK
SALADS	KITCHEN WISDOM

A REVOLUTIONARY APPROACH TO FOOD AND FITNESS

TASTE of LIFE

JULIE STAFFORD

THE DIET THAT SAVED A LIFE

Julie and Bruce Stafford thought they had the perfect life and family until, out-of-the-blue, 30 year-old Bruce, who had never missed a day's work through illness in his life, was struck down by cancer.

As Bruce's health steadily deteriorated, Julie decided to investigate the link between diet and disease. She came up with an eating plan based on the principle of low-fat, salt-free and sugar-free foods but applied it to inventive, delicious and mouth-watering recipes. The result? A miraculous recovery. Within two weeks Bruce's health improved and now he is completely cured.

Julie Stafford shows you how to eat like a gourmet and be healthy too. TASTE OF LIFE is truly a revolutionary, life-sustaining breakthrough.

0 7221 8105 1   HEALTH/COOKERY   £3.50

ROBYN WILSON

FISH

The complete A–Z of over a hundred irresistible fish and shellfish, covering everything you need to know about buying, preparing and cooking this most versatile and appetizing food – for beginner and expert alike.

FISH for your health
– Halve your chances of a heart attack
– Increase your resistance to arthritis, migraine headaches, multiple sclerosis, eczema, breast cancer and high blood pressure
– Increase your brain power

FISH for your figure
– Lose weight with low calorie fish
– Keep your skin supple, your eyes bright and your hair shiny
– Reduce the cholesterol level in your diet

FISH for your sex life
– Enhance your potency, fertility and libido

FISH – the ultimate guide to a new lifestyle of health and fitness.

0 7474 0037 7   NON-FICTION   £2.50

Howard & Maschler
O·N F·O·O·D

Elizabeth Jane Howard & Fay Maschler

'A joy to read, witty and shrewd'
Daily Mail

With wit, insight and an acute grasp of life's vicissitudes, Elizabeth Jane Howard and Fay Maschler, two well-known and prominent writers, have combined their culinary enthusiasm to produce a mouth-watering collection of recipes which are specially chosen to complement the varied occasions that life presents: A house-moving supper; a winter picnic; a seductive meal for a lover; dinner to enliven dull guests; food to cheer the abandoned man; a budget dinner party; a ladies' lunch.

For cooks of all levels of ability and lifestyle – those with limited resources, pressures of time, the rich, the put-upon, the eccentric – this is a stimulating, down-to-earth, inspiring cookbook which is as life-enhancing as the recipes are delicious.

'Two women with vast experience of family life behind them, celebrate both the strength of female friendship and the sustaining female world of food and comfort' *The Times*

0 7474 0196 9   COOKERY   £3.99

Mary Berry

BUFFETS

The perfect guide to buffets for all occasions

Preparing a buffet for a dozen people or more can be a daunting prospect. Everybody wonders what to make, how much to make and what is that magic ingredient which turns it into a meal to remember.

In BUFFETS, Mary Berry's practical advice, excellent menu suggestions and over 200 mouth watering recipes cover every possible occasion, providing invaluable help and encouragement to experienced and not-so-experienced cooks alike.

Including essential tips on planning and organization, hire of equipment, table decoration, presentation, garnishing and choice of drinks, the recipes are divided into such themes as, Finger Foods, Summer Buffets, Winter Buffets, Victorian Buffets, Scottish Highland Buffets, American Buffets, Italian Buffets and Indian Buffets. Each delicious section includes soups and starters, main courses, vegetables and salads, puddings, party breads and biscuits.

BUFFETS – the ideal companion to all help-yourself parties:

Also by Mary Berry in Sphere Books:

FAST CAKES
MORE FAST CAKES
FAST DESSERTS
FAST SUPPERS
FRUIT FARE

FAST STARTERS, SOUPS
AND SALADS
FEED YOUR FAMILY THE
HEALTHIER WAY
CHOCOLATE DELIGHTS

0 7221 1640 3   COOKERY   £3.99

A selection of bestsellers from SPHERE

FICTION

JUBILEE: THE POPPY CHRONICLES 1	Claire Rayner	£3.50 ☐
DAUGHTERS	Suzanne Goodwin	£3.50 ☐
REDCOAT	Bernard Cornwell	£3.50 ☐
WHEN DREAMS COME TRUE	Emma Blair	£3.50 ☐
THE LEGACY OF HEOROT	Niven/Pournelle/Barnes	£3.50 ☐

FILM AND TV TIE-IN

BUSTER	Colin Shindler	£2.99 ☐
COMING TOGETHER	Alexandra Hine	£2.99 ☐
RUN FOR YOUR LIFE	Stuart Collins	£2.99 ☐
BLACK FOREST CLINIC	Peter Heim	£2.99 ☐
INTIMATE CONTACT	Jacqueline Osborne	£2.50 ☐

NON-FICTION

BARE-FACED MESSIAH	Russell Miller	£3.99 ☐
THE COCHIN CONNECTION	Alison and Brian Milgate	£3.50 ☐
HOWARD & MASCHLER ON FOOD	Elizabeth Jane Howard and Fay Maschler	£3.99 ☐
FISH	Robyn Wilson	£2.50 ☐
THE SACRED VIRGIN AND THE HOLY WHORE	Anthony Harris	£3.50 ☐

All Sphere books are available at your local bookshop or newsagent, or can be ordered direct from the publisher. Just tick the titles you want and fill in the form below.

Name _____

Address _____

Write to Sphere Books, Cash Sales Department, P.O. Box 11, Falmouth, Cornwall TR10 9EN

Please enclose a cheque or postal order to the value of the cover price plus:

UK: 60p for the first book, 25p for the second book and 15p for each additional book ordered to a maximum charge of £1.90.

OVERSEAS & EIRE: £1.25 for the first book, 75p for the second book and 28p for each subsequent title ordered.

BFPO: 60p for the first book, 25p for the second book plus 15p per copy for the next 7 books, thereafter 9p per book.

Sphere Books reserve the right to show new retail prices on covers which may differ from those previously advertised in the text elsewhere, and to increase postal rates in accordance with the P.O.